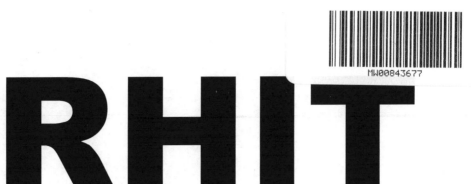

# RHIT
# Exam
# Practice Questions

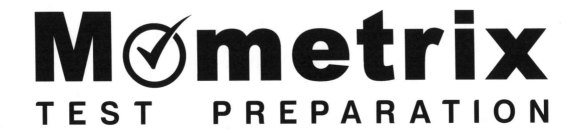

# DEAR FUTURE EXAM SUCCESS STORY

First of all, **THANK YOU** for purchasing Mometrix study materials!

Second, congratulations! You are one of the few determined test-takers who are committed to doing whatever it takes to excel on your exam. **You have come to the right place.** We developed these practice tests with one goal in mind: to deliver you the best possible approximation of the questions you will see on test day.

Standardized testing is one of the biggest obstacles on your road to success, which only increases the importance of doing well in the high-pressure, high-stakes environment of test day. Your results on this test could have a significant impact on your future, and these practice tests will give you the repetitions you need to build your familiarity and confidence with the test content and format to help you achieve your full potential on test day.

### Your success is our success

**We would love to hear from you!** If you would like to share the story of your exam success or if you have any questions or comments in regard to our products, please contact us at **800-673-8175** or **support@mometrix.com**.

Thanks again for your business and we wish you continued success!

Sincerely,
The Mometrix Test Preparation Team

# TABLE OF CONTENTS

# Practice Test #1

**1. A hospital has a base MS-DRG of $5040.00 and the following adjustments:**

Value based purchasing (VBP): (-$5.06)
Disproportionate share hospital (DSH): +$128.56
Indirect medical education (IME): +$486.22
Readmission adjustment: (-$1.08)

**What is the new base operating MS-DRG (subject to case mix)?**

a. $5660.92
b. $5651.78
c. $5650.52
d. $5648.64

**2. In which PPS is the RUG-IV group classification system used?**

a. Acute care hospital
b. SNF
c. Children's hospital
d. Home health agency

**3. Which of the following is required of a Health Insurance Portability and Accountability Act (HIPAA) covered entity that experiences a security breach that resulted in unauthorized access of PHI of 650 individuals?**

a. Notify the individuals only within 30 days.
b. Notify the individuals within 30 days and provide an annual report to HHS.
c. Notify the individuals, HHS, and local news media within 60 days.
d. Notify the individual, HHS, and local news media within 30 days.

**4. Which of the following allows healthcare organizations and pharmacies to communicate drug-related information efficiently?**

a. SNOMED CT
b. NDC
c. RxNorm
d. LOINC

**5. Under which circumstance may it be acceptable to document a discharge note only instead of a full discharge summary?**

a. Uncomplicated stay of fewer than 48 hours.
b. Uncomplicated stay of fewer than 24 hours.
c. All stays for childbirth.
d. Under no circumstances

**6. In addition to the CDT code for removal of a tooth, what other information is required?**

a. No other information
b. Tooth type
c. Date of last dental cleaning
d. Tooth number

1

**7. A patient with malignant neoplasm of the head of the pancreas (C25.0) is admitted to the hospital for management of pain related to the malignancy (G89.3). The patient has anemia due to antineoplastic chemotherapy (D64.81) for which the patient has been receiving ongoing treatment but is presently stable. How would these diagnostic codes be sequenced (first to last)?**

    a. C25.0, D64.81, and G89.3
    b. G89.3, C25.0, and D64.81
    c. G89.3, D64.81, and C25.0
    d. D64.81, C25.0, and G89.3

**8. Accreditation surveys by The Joint Commission take place on a minimum cycle of every:**

    a. year
    b. 2 years
    c. 3 years
    d. 4 years

**9. Medicare will waive an organization's need for a compliance audit if it is appropriately accredited by granting which of the following?**

    a. Registered status
    b. Deemed status
    c. Certification
    d. Conditional compliance

**10. When a patient has a gallbladder surgically removed and the specimen is examined in the laboratory and a report is generated that describes the gross appearance as well as the microscopic findings, this report is referred to as a(n):**

    a. pathology report.
    b. operative report.
    c. laboratory report.
    d. consultation report.

**11. If a hospital has 200 licensed beds available and 150 of those beds are filled with patients, the current occupancy rate for the day is:**

    a. 150%
    b. 100%
    c. 75%
    d. 50%

**12. Under the IRF PPS, if a patient is discharged from a rehabilitation facility on July 16, by which date is data transmission of the discharge patient assessment instrument (PAI) to CMS considered late?**

    a. July 26
    b. August 4
    c. August 12
    d. August 16

13. Community Hospital has allocated funds for additional staffing for the emergency department and has asked the HIM department to gather statistics regarding the average wait time for the previous 6 months. Over this time period, the emergency department has adopted a number of measures to increase efficiency. Based on the average wait times, which time period has shown the least progress and may most benefit from additional staffing?

Average Wait Time in Emergency Department in Minutes

| TIME | Jan | Feb | Mar | April | May | June |
|------|-----|-----|-----|-------|-----|------|
| 7AM-12N | 44 | 43 | 42 | 38 | 39 | 40 |
| 12N-7PM | 58 | 56 | 48 | 40 | 35 | 32 |
| 7PM-12M | 38 | 36 | 40 | 31 | 28 | 30 |
| 12M-7AM | 34 | 30 | 24 | 25 | 29 | 26 |

    a. 7AM-12N
    b. 12N-7PM
    c. 7PM-12M
    d. 12M-7AM

14. A staff member of a healthcare facility has authorized access to ePHI but has given 2 weeks' notice of intent to resign. What procedure must be implemented when the person resigns?
    a. Workforce clearance
    b. Termination
    c. Access modification
    d. Password management

15. If a hospital with 300 licensed and available beds has an average length of stay (ALOS) of 5 days, how many patients could the hospital serve in a 30-day period?
    a. 1200
    b. 1500
    c. 1800
    d. 2000

16. Which of the following is the standard format that is used by hospitals and other institutional providers to transmit health claims electronically to CMS?
    a. 837I
    b. 837P
    c. UB-04
    d. CMS-1500

17. Patients in acute care facilities usually do not stay more than:
    a. 5 days
    b. 15 days
    c. 20 days
    d. 30 days

**18. Which department in an acute care facility is considered an outpatient department rather than inpatient?**

    a. Ob-gyn
    b. ED
    c. Medical
    d. Pediatrics

**19. If a patient is admitted to an acute care facility at 11:50 PM on May 2 and discharged at 7 AM on May 6, what is the LOS?**

    a. 2 days
    b. 3 days
    c. 4 days
    d. 5 days

**20. HL7 refers to:**

    a. Health Level 7.
    b. Health Label 7.
    c. Hardware Level 7
    d. Hitech Level 7.

**21. HIPAA was passed by Congress in what year?**

    a. 1966
    b. 1976
    c. 1986
    d. 1996

**22. According to HIPAA's Privacy Rule regarding authorization forms, which of the following is *not* a required element?**

    a. Expiration date
    b. Consent for treatment
    c. The information that may be disclosed.
    d. How the information will be used.

**23. In the tables in the relational database, what is the primary key and what is the foreign key?**

**Table 1 (Parent table)**

| Emp_No | Last_Name | First_Name | Gender |
|--------|-----------|------------|--------|
| 001 | Jones | James | M |
| 002 | Evans | Sarah | F |
| 003 | Smythe | James | M |

**Table 2 (Child table)**

| Emp_No | Work_Status |
|--------|-------------|
| 001 | Part-time |
| 002 | Full-time |
| 003 | Part-time |

a. Emp_No is the primary key in table 1 and Emp_No is the foreign key in table 2.
b. Emp_No is the primary key in table 1 and Work_Status is the foreign key in table 2.
c. Last_Name is the primary key in table 1 and Emp_No is the foreign key in table 2.
d. Last-Name is the primary key in table 1 and Work_Status is the foreign key in table 2.

**24. The Security Rule of HIPAA applies to:**

a. all PHI.
b. personally identifiable information.
c. PHI in paper form only.
d. ePHI only.

**25. During planning for implementation of a new EHR, the HIM department plans user acceptance testing (UAT) to determine if the end users are willing and able to use the new equipment and applications as intended. The first step to analyzing end-user acceptance is to:**

a. design test cases and testing plan.
b. identify different acceptance scenarios.
c. determine the basic system and organization requirements.
d. describe the severity levels of the testing plan.

**26. The maximum value of a byte in terms of bits is:**

a. 32
b. 64
c. 128
d. 256

**27. In a relational database, the data are separated into defined logical groups by:**

a. tables.
b. fields
c. records.
d. characters.

28. Although a healthcare organization has no formal policy regarding personal use of computers or the Internet, the administration believes that the staff "understand" restrictions on use and has asked the HIM department to monitor employee emails and Internet use to determine if staff members are divulging PHI or writing negative statements about the organization. What is the appropriate response to the administration?

    a. The administration must first establish written policies regarding computer/Internet use.
    b. Information gained from tracking emails and Internet use can be used to develop policies.
    c. A written policy is not necessary if there is general understanding of restrictions.
    d. The organization cannot legally limit or monitor employees' personal use of computers/Internet.

29. If an acute care hospital invested in new diagnostic equipment at a cost of $520,000 and showed a benefit of $825,000 at the end of the year, what is the return on investment (ROI) (rounded to the nearest whole number)?

    a. 31%
    b. 59%
    c. 63%
    d. 158%

30. When a patient is admitted to a hospital, what should the registration clerk do to ensure that a duplicate record is not created for a patient who is already registered in the system?

    a. Ask the patient about prior admissions.
    c. Assign a new ID number.
    b. Check the master patient index (MPI).
    d. Telephone the records department.

31. According to AHIMA's minimum retention schedule, how long should diagnostic images, such as x-rays, be retained?

    a. 5 years
    b. 10 years
    c. Permanently
    d. 20 years

**32.** The HIM department of a newly expanded hospital must hire coders to keep up with billing as productivity has slowed with institution of ICD-10-CM/PCS, and some staff members have retired. Average number of records completed per hour:

| Category | Average coding per hour |
|---|---|
| Inpatients | 2.5 |
| Ambulatory surgery patients | 3.5 |
| ED visits | 7 |
| Ancillary services (testing, laboratory) | 10 |

**The additional coding needs per week are for:**

- 500 inpatient discharge charts
- 420 ambulatory surgery charts
- 840 ED charts
- 800 ancillary services

**Assuming that coders work a 40-hour week, how many FTE coders are needed to fulfill these coding needs?**
   a.   10
   b.   13
   c.   22
   d.   36

**33.** An example of a primary purpose for an electronic health record is:
   a.   evidence in litigation.
   b.   clinical research.
   c.   patient care management.
   d.   allocation of resources.

**34.** Following a clinical pertinence review, one physician was found to have completed history and physical exam documentations 3 to 5 days after the physician actually conducted the history and physical examinations for 20 patients. Which of the following quality characteristics of data quality management has been violated?
   a.   Data accuracy
   b.   Data granularity
   c.   Data relevancy
   d.   Data currency

**35.** The process through which data are archived is referred to as:
   a.   data warehousing.
   b.   data collection.
   c.   data analysis.
   d.   data applications.

**36.** If paper health records are filed using terminal digit filing and a patient's health record is numbered 44-62-10, in which section will the chart be filed?
   a.   Section 44
   b.   Section 62
   c.   Section 10
   d.   Either Section 10 or Section 44

**37. Which accrediting organization accredits a wide range of healthcare facilities and organizations, including acute care hospitals, children's hospitals, psychiatric institutions, rehabilitation centers, clinical laboratories, long-term care facilities, and home health agencies?**

a. NCQA
b. AAAHC
c. CARF
d. TJC

**38. In a paper chart filing system, an outguide is used to:**

a. label sections in the filing system.
b. track records that have been checked out.
c. develop an index of filed records.
d. label the outside of records with identifying information.

**39. Which of the following is a *technical* safeguard of the Security Standards in HIPAA?**

a. Delegation of security responsibilities
b. Retaining computer backups offsite
c. Encrypting and decrypting
d. Restricting access to data

**40. If using SQL to query a relational database with the headings as in the table below, what is the correct query for a list of patient IDs and patient names for patients who attended the Well-Baby clinic only?**

**Clinic_Patients**

| Pat_ID | Last_Name | First_Name | Clinic | Ad_Date |
|--------|-----------|------------|----------|------------|
| 001 | Evans | Maria | WellBaby | 01/06/2016 |
| 002 | Locke | James | HIV_AIDS | 12/03/2015 |

a. SELECT Pat_ID, Last_Name, First_Name, Clinic FROM Clinic_Patients WHERE Clinic = 'WellBaby'
b. Pat-ID, Last_Name, First_Name, WellBaby FROM Clinic_Patients
c. SELECT Pat_ID, Last_Name, First_Name, Wellbaby FROM Clinic_Patients WHERE = 'WellBaby'
d. SELECT Pat_ID, Last_Name, First_Name, Clinic FROM Clinic_Patients WHERE Clinic = <> 'WellBaby'

**41. Which of the following types of patient data misuse occur if a physician cannot remember his or her new password and uses another staff person's password to access data about a patient?**

a. Identify theft
b. Privacy violation
c. Security breach
d. Unauthorized access

**42. The PHR differs from the EHR in that the PHR is:**
a. controlled by the physician.
b. controlled by the individual.
c. not governed by rules about privacy or confidentiality.
d. contains only information from the individual.

**43. The repair costs associated with improper computer equipment use have resulted in overtime payments of approximately 40 hours per month at a cost of $125 per hour. The HIM director proposes training additional staff persons to carry out the repairs in order to decrease overtime to an average of 10 hours per month, but the cost for materials is $400, the instructor is $3000, and staff costs for release time are $2000 for each of 6 staff members. What would be the cost benefit of this training in the first year?**
a. There would be cost benefit of $29,600.
b. There would be cost benefit of $39,600.
c. There would be cost benefit of $44,600.
d. There would be no cost benefit.

**44. The HIM department must purchase or lease new hardware to replace an outdated system. The HIM department has identified four potential vendors through attendance at conferences, research of publications, and recommendations from other organizations. The next step in the vendor selection process is to:**
a. develop a contract.
b. narrow the vendors to two.
c. send a request for information (RFI).
d. send a request for proposal (RFP).

**45. When conducting trending analysis of data in a run chart, a *run* occurs with:**
a. ≥ 7 consecutive data points in either ascending or descending order with ≥ 21 total data points or ≥ 6 with fewer than 21 total data points.
b. up and down variation forming a sawtooth pattern with 14 successive data points.
c. data point unrelated to other points in the chart.
d. ≥ 7 data consecutive data points all above or all below the median.

**46. The laboratory in an acute hospital has begun sending automated alerts by instant messaging to physicians for all abnormal lab results rather than telephoning to try to improve response rate. However, studies show that many alerts are ignored, and response time has only slightly improved. In order to improve response time, the best method is likely to:**
a. reset parameters for alerts for all tests.
b. advise disciplinary action against physicians.
c. reward physicians for improving response time.
d. discontinue the automated system of alerts.

**47. Prior to upgrading to a new EHR system, the HIM department conducts workflow analysis to ensure the EHR integrates well into the clinical workflow. Which of the following steps should be taken first?**

a. Determine future requirements.
b. Determine benefits of the upgrade.
c. Assess the current status.
d. Assess utilization of physical space and equipment.

**48. While an acute care hospital has instituted barcodes on patient ID bracelets and medications in order to decrease medication errors in order to comply with National Patient Safety Goals, a survey finds that common practice is to copy the barcodes and place them on the medicine cart for scanning so that nurses can prepare a number of different medicines at one time to deliver later to patients. Which of the following statements about this practice is correct?**

a. This practice is acceptable if the medicines are delivered within 1 hour.
b. This practice is acceptable only in emergencies.
c. This practice is acceptable if ID is again checked at the point of care.
d. This practice is never acceptable as ID is not at the point of care.

**49. To ensure that a hospital's EHR aligns with the CMS EHR Incentive Program, it is necessary to:**

a. be 80% compliant with CMS required criteria to demonstrate Meaningful Use.
b. be 100% compliant with CMS required criteria to demonstrate Meaningful Use.
c. apply for certification through CMS regardless of compliance.
d. pay a fee for certification to participate in the program.

**50. Which of the following is the primary purpose for reviewing the audit trails of EHRs?**

a. To determine if the EHR has undergone unauthorized access.
b. To determine if the EHR is storing data properly.
c. To determine if the patient has been advised of privacy/security regulations.
d. To determine if the EHR data has been entered in a timely manner.

**51. The purpose of the compliance plans established by the Office of the Inspector General (OIG) is to ensure that:**

a. patients' rights are respected.
b. organizations switch from paper records to EHRs.
c. organizations bill for services properly.
d. patient records are retained for specified periods of time.

52. If a patient was admitted to the hospital for occlusion of the right femoral artery and underwent an open surgical procedure in which the right femoral artery was dilated with a drug-coated balloon and a drug-eluting stent placed in the lumen of the artery, the correct ICD-10-PCS code is:

    a. 047K0D1 Dilation of right femoral artery with intraluminal device using drug-coated balloon, open approach
    b. 047K041 Dilation of right femoral artery with drug-eluting intraluminal device using drug-coated balloon, open approach
    c. 047K0Z1 Dilation of right femoral artery using drug-coated balloon, open approach
    d. 047K3D1 Dilation of the right femoral artery with intraluminal device using drug-coated balloon, percutaneous approach

53. In order to avoid medical records being classified as delinquent, within what period following discharge of patients from the hospital must records be completed, including inclusion of the final diagnosis?

    a. 48 hours
    b. 7 days
    c. 21 days
    d. 30 days

54. Which of the following ICD-10-CM codes is non-covered by Medicare for all lab national coverage determinations (NCDs)?

    a. Z00.01 Encounter for general adult medical examination with abnormal findings
    b. G93.3 Postviral fatigue syndrome
    c. N39.44 Nocturnal enuresis
    d. R00.0 Tachycardia, unspecified

55. If creating a data dictionary to correspond to the table below, what would the data dictionary define?

Patient Information

| ID # | Last_Name | First_Name | Gender | Birthdate |
|------|-----------|-----------|--------|-----------|
| 001 | Statler | Josiah | M | 12/16/1944 |
| 002 | Manley | Jane | F | 05/29/1929 |

    a. ID #, last name, first name, gender, and birthdate
    b. field name, data length, type of data, and order of fields
    c. table name, field name, type of data, and order of fields
    d. table name, field name, length, and type of data

56. If the HIM director is planning to make changes in order to increase efficiency and wants to begin by carrying out a gap analysis, the first step in gap analysis is to identify:

    a. best practices.
    b. key individuals.
    c. barriers.
    d. timeline.

**57. In a relational database, what are the three types of possible anomalies?**

a. Deviation, update, and insertion
b. Update, insertion, and deletion
c. Insertion, translation, and deviation
d. Translocation, insertion, and deletion

**58. If two computers and a server were stolen because the door to the room with the equipment was left ajar, which type of security measure is insufficient?**

a. Management practices
b. Technical measures
c. Physical safeguards
d. Hazard measures

**59. How far away from a healthcare organization should a "warm" site with patient data be located?**

a. Within 5 miles
b. More than 20 miles
c. At least 50 miles
d. At least 100 miles

**60. Which of the following types of incidents would usually result in the involvement of a law enforcement agency?**

a. A computer virus infects a server.
b. An employee is suspected of identity theft.
c. An employee enters data into the record of the wrong patient.
d. An employee shares a password with another employee.

**61. Prior to the installation of a new computer system, the HIM department conducts volume testing. The purpose of volume testing is to:**

a. identify the upper limits at which the computer system can function adequately.
b. determine how many computer stations are needed for the system.
c. determine the processing speed of the computers.
d. identify flaws in the design of the computer system.

**62. When training new staff members in the HIM department about data flow within a healthcare organization, the best method is likely to:**

a. present the information in a lecture.
b. provide a data-flow diagram.
c. carry out a question and answer session.
d. conduct one-on-one training.

63. Community Hospital carried out a clinical pertinence reivew by randomly pulling and reviewing approximately 10% of records from each of 5 clinical departments to assess completion rates in order to begin preparation for accreditation. There are approximately 600 physicians serving the hospital. The hospital administration would like to target review of documentation procedures where it will be most effective, aiming for at least 95% completion rates across the board. Based on the initial findings, which department or departments are most in need of review of procedures?

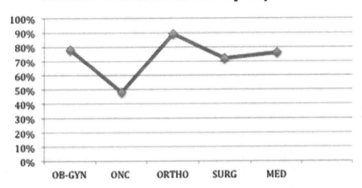

Clinical Pertinence Review by Department

a. ONC, SURG, and MED
b. ONC
c. All departments
d. Data are insufficient.

64. Physicians and other staff members at County Hospital are increasingly utilizing mobile devices and want to access patient records and enter data over the Internet via the devices. The HIM department is assisting in the development of a mobile device policy. All of the following are critical measures to include *except*:

a. establishment of a VPN.
b. installation of remote disabling/wiping.
c. security/privacy training.
d. insurance policy against loss.

65. The County Hospital administration is considering transitioning to cloud storage and has asked the HIM department to assess vendors and gather information. Which of the following is the most important initial issue to consider?

a. initial and ongoing costs
b. reputation of vendor
c. compliance with regulations
d. interoperability

66. When conducting an audit of narcotic prescriptions in the emergency department, the HIM director notes that one physician had ordered 4 times more narcotics than any other physician in the department over a 1-month period, with multiple prescriptions to some individuals who returned frequently to the emergency department. What is the most appropriate action?

  a.  No action is needed.
  b.  Notify the police.
  c.  Ask the physician for an explanation.
  d.  Alert the administration.

67. Which of the following HCPCS level II codes is used when filing a Medicare claim for durable medical equipment, such as a bedside commode?

  a.  D codes
  b.  E codes
  c.  L codes
  d.  P codes

68. As part of the review process for short-stay (fewer than 2 midnights) inpatients, the Quality Improvement Organization (QIO) acting for CMS will pull how many short-stay inpatient records from small and large hospitals to determine medical necessity?

  a.  5 from small and 10 from large
  b.  10 from small and 20 from large
  c.  20 from small and 50 from large
  d.  50 from small and 100 from large

69. Under ICD-10-CM, unspecified codes are used when:

  a.  sufficient information about the condition is not yet available.
  b.  an injury is accidental.
  c.  the patient has a combination of conditions.
  d.  attempting to simplify coding.

70. Which of the following is a data set or initiative that supports collecting data from emergency departments in hospitals?

  a.  ORYX
  b.  HEDIS
  c.  DEEDS
  d.  NHIN

71. When reporting other diagnoses or conditions beyond the primary diagnosis for UHDDS, which of the following is correct?

  a.  Report all other conditions and diagnoses.
  b.  Report acute conditions but not chronic conditions.
  d.  Include previous diagnoses.
  c.  Report diagnoses associated with current health services.

**72. Which part of Medicare coverage includes Medicare Advantage Plans?**

    a. Part A
    b. Part B
    c. Part C
    d. Parts A and B

**73. County Hospital has received an administrative request from a law enforcement official for copies of a patient's records related to a criminal proceeding. According to HIPAA's Privacy Rule, what three criteria must be met before information is disclosed?**

    a. Relevance, specificity, and identifiable information necessary
    b. Reason, identifying information, and specificity
    c. Relevance, identifying information, and specificity
    d. Reason, relevance, and identifiable information necessary

**74. Which workload (data) distribution techniques are used with a distributed database?**

    a. Analysis, integration, and fragmentation
    b. Analysis, allocation, and integration
    c. Fragmentation, analysis, and integration
    d. Fragmentation, allocation, and replication

**75. If a hospital is among the 25% of hospitals with the highest rates of hospital-acquired conditions (HACs), what percentage reduction in payment will the CMS impose?**

    a. 0.5%
    b. 1%
    c. 2%
    d. 3%

**76. A patient's primary diagnosis reads "Renal cell carcinoma of the upper pole of left kidney, stage 1, grade 2." Which of the following ICD-10-CM codes should be applied?**

| |
|---|
| C64 Malignant neoplasm of kidney, except renal pelvis |
| C64.1 Malignant neoplasm of right kidney, except renal pelvis. |
| C64.2 Malignant neoplasm of left kidney, except renal pelvis. |
| C64.9 Malignant neoplasm of unspecified kidney, except renal pelvis. |
| C65 Malignant neoplasm of renal pelvis |
| C65.1 Malignant neoplasm of right renal pelvis. |
| C65.2 Malignant neoplasm of left renal pelvis. |
| C65.9 Malignant neoplasm of unspecified renal pelvis. |
| C68 Malignant neoplasm of other and unspecified urinary organs |
| C68.9 Malignant neoplasm of urinary organ, unspecified. |

    a. C64.2
    b. C65.2
    c. C65.9
    d. C68.9

**77. The three criteria that electronic signatures must meet when used for medical records are:**

    a. user authentication, non-duplication, and confirmation.
    b. confirmation, nonrepudiation, and user authentication.
    c. message integrity, nonrepudiation, and user authentication.
    d. message integrity, non-duplication, and user authentication.

**78. If, during a system upgrade, a system failure results in corrupted data, the immediate response should be to:**

    a. revert to backup.
    b. correct the data.
    c. determine the exact cause.
    d. consult with experts.

**79. A patient was hospitalized as an inpatient in an acute care hospital under Medicare A from March 7 to March 15. If Medicare is to pay for skilled nursing facility care, within how many days after discharge must the patient be admitted to the skilled nursing facility?**

    a. 14
    b. 21
    c. 30
    d. 60

**80. The purpose of an Advance Beneficiary Notice is to:**

    a. make decisions about end-of-life care.
    b. notify patients that they have been overcharged for a service.
    c. notify patients that services they received were not covered by Medicare.
    d. notify patients that a service may not be covered by Medicare.

**81. According to the charge description master (CDM; also called the chargemaster), if a patient was hospitalized in the ICU for 3 days and had hourly telemetry for 24 hours, 4 ECGs, and cardioversion, how much would be charged to payers?**

| # | Charge code | Item | Price | CPT | Rev code |
|---|---|---|---|---|---|
| 001 | 10006873 | Telemetry Hourly | 300.00 | 99220 | 762 |
| 002 | 10021988 | ICU room charge, Normal | 9112.00 | | 200 |
| 003 | 31068216 | Cardioversion, Defib. | 1820.00 | 92960 | 480 |
| 004 | 31072831 | ECG w/o interp | 765.00 | 93005 | 730 |

    a. $11,997.00
    b. $19,952.00
    c. $27,590.00
    d. $39,396.00

**82. According to the six stages of the revenue cycle, after services are provided, the next stage involves:**

    a. establishing charges.
    b. documenting services.
    c. submitting claim for services.
    d. prepare bill for services.

**83.** When utilizing a *charge explosion* system for the charge master, five different chargeable items that are part of one service would be entered into the system under:

    a.  one code.
    b.  two codes.
    c.  four codes.
    d.  five codes.

**84.** If a claim for outpatient service is billed to Medicare and outpatient code edits (OCE) result in a claim-level disposition of *suspension*, what must the healthcare provider do?

    a.  File an appeal with Medicare.
    b.  Provide requested information.
    c.  Correct problems prior to resubmission.
    d.  Correct the claim prior to resubmission.

**85.** A healthcare provider applies multiple codes, resulting in multiple claims, for a service that should have been covered by one code and one claim. This is an example of:

    a.  upcoding.
    b.  downcoding.
    c.  double billing.
    d.  unbundling.

**86.** If the hospital administrator wants to compare the caseloads of different oncologists on the staff and asks the HIM director to prepare a report, the most appropriate place to find that data is the:

    a.  EHRs.
    b.  physician index.
    c.  cancer registry.
    d.  disease registry.

**87.** A well-known local politician is hospitalized, and specific information about the politician's physical exam, diagnosis, and treatment is leaked to a local newspaper, suggesting that the information came from a healthcare provider. The best method to determine who leaked the information is to:

    a.  provide a reward for information.
    b.  ask the newspaper who provided the information.
    c.  conduct an audit trail.
    d.  ask the police to conduct an investigation.

**88.** County Hospital wants to decrease the rate of readmissions by providing high-risk patients with case managers. The best method to identify these patients is to:

    a.  use software application to mine data regarding risk factors from the EHRs.
    b.  ask unit supervisors to notify the case manager of potential cases.
    c.  conduct patient surveys, asking if they want case managers.
    d.  use software to trigger alerts of patients hospitalized for more than 3 days.

89. The hospital has established a facility-based trauma registry, and a patient who is to be added to the registry was first admitted in May of 2015. The patient was the 20th patient added to the registry that year, and this was the patient's first incidence of trauma. The correct accession number is:
    a. 15-0020-01
    b. 20-0020-01
    c. 2015-20-01
    d. 15-20-0001

90. If a patient was hospitalized for 4 days and then discharged but readmitted 6 days later for a 3-day stay, does the patient need to have any history and physical exam completed for the second hospitalization?
    a. No, no history and physical is needed.
    b. Yes, a complete history and physical exam must be done.
    c. Yes, an interval history and physical exam must be done.
    d. Yes, but only if the patient is readmitted for a different problem.

91. According to CMS, the three key components when selecting the correct level of E/M services (not including visits for counseling and/or coordination of care) are history, _____, and decision making.
    a. examination.
    b. recommendation.
    c. documentation.
    d. reason for referral.

92. An example of a finding associated with a *qualitative* review of an EHR is:
    a. electronic signature missing from a progress report.
    b. pathology report of surgical specimen not in the record.
    c. dressing change not documented for one day.
    d. results of an ordered CBC are not in the record.

93. A patient with poorly controlled COPD and diabetes mellitus required five different hospitalizations in 1 year. The patient's care is covered by Medicare A and secondary insurance. According to CMS guidelines, how many benefit periods did the patient have?

| Admission Date | Discharge Date |
| --- | --- |
| May 1 | May 15 |
| July 2 | July 8 |
| August 10 | August 30 |
| September 18 | September 22 |
| October 10 | October 14 |

    a. One
    b. Two
    c. Three
    d. Five

**94.** County Hospital experienced a flood when a nearby river overflowed during a severe rainstorm, inundating the records room located in the basement and saturating a large volume of records. The best salvage method is to:
   a. separate the papers in the records and air dry.
   b. separate the papers in the records and apply heat and fans.
   c. keep the records intact and freeze them.
   d. separate the papers in the records and freeze them.

**95.** Which of the following is the standard data code set under HIPAA for pharmacy transactions involving drugs and biologics and is included in Medicare D data?
   a. NANDA
   b. NDC
   c. SNOMED CT
   d. CDT

**96.** With ICD-10-CM, injuries are grouped by:
   a. system.
   b. category of injury.
   c. severity of injury.
   d. body part.

**97.** According to ICD-10-PCS, if a patient undergoes a thrombectomy to remove a clot from the leg, which of the following is the root operation for this surgical procedure?
   a. Extraction
   b. Excision
   c. Extirpation
   d. Removal

**98.** As part of denials management, if coding has been missing for some services because physicians frequently forget to document bedside procedures, such as wound care, the best solution may be to:
   a. provide coders access to account charges.
   b. institute back-end editing.
   c. send out reminders to physicians.
   d. provide better training for coders.

**99.** When an enterprise-wide master patient index (MPI) fails to link two medical files for a patient who has been treated at two participating organizations and the patient ends up with two identifiers in the MPI, this type of error is a(n):
   a. duplication.
   b. distortion.
   c. overlay.
   d. overlap.

**100. If a hospital has an average of 450 discharges every month and the number of delinquent records for 1 month is 126, what is the delinquency rate for the month?**

a. 36%
b. 28%
c. 76%
d. 42%

**101. If utilizing an unlisted procedure code for CPT coding for a surgical procedure, what further submission is required?**

a. No further submission required.
b. Pathology report
c. Operative report
d. Discharge summary

**102. A patient was scheduled for an outpatient mastectomy because of a small cancerous lesion and planned to have reconstruction done immediately after breast removal. Possible modifiers include:**

LT, Left side.
53, Procedure discontinued.
52, Reduced services.

**The operative report describes the procedures as "complete left mastectomy with insertion of breast prosthesis. Nipple reconstruction began but discontinued when patient became severely hypotensive." What procedure codes are indicated?**

| CPT/HCPCS Code | Description of Procedure |
|---|---|
| 50230 | Mastectomy for gynecomastia |
| 19301 | Mastectomy, partial (e.g. lumpectomy, tylectomy, quadrantectomy, segmentectomy) |
| 19303 | Mastectomy, simple, complete. |
| 19304 | Mastectomy, subcutaneous |
| 19340 | Immediate insertion of breast prosthesis following mastopexy, mastectomy, or in reconstruction. |
| 19350 | Nipple/areola reconstruction |
| 19357 | Breast reconstruction, immediate or delayed, with tissue expander, including subsequent expansion |

a. 19303-LT, 19340-LT, 19350-LT-52-LT
b. 19303-LT, 19340 LT, 19350-LT-52
c. 19304-LT, 19340, 19350-LT-53.
d. 19303-LT, 19340-LT, 19350-53-LT

**103. A patient had a skin tag removed on March 1 and returned to the same physician on March 3 for a laceration repair unrelated to the first surgery. How many days total would the patient be covered under the Medicare's global surgical package for the minor surgical procedures?**

a. 10
b. 11
c. 13
d. 22

**104.** An 8-year-old child is brought to the emergency department by a non-related family friend after the child fell and complained of leg pain, but the child walked into the emergency department. The parents could not be reached. Which of the following is appropriate before the parents are reached?

    a. A medical screening exam only should be conducted.
    b. The family friend can sign consent form for tests and treatment.
    c. Because this is an emergency, the physician can order tests and treatment.
    d. A court order should be obtained before providing care.

**105.** All of the following are critical roles that the HIM department plays in data standardization *except*:

    a. Identifying key elements requiring standardization.
    b. Carrying out clinical document improvement functions.
    c. Ensuring national data standards are in use in the organization.
    d. Ensuring that data support financial goals of the organization.

**106.** Considering the domains of quality management, which of the following refers to the purpose of the collection of data?

    a. Collection
    b. Application
    c. Analysis
    d. Warehousing

**107.** Which of the following can trigger the requirement for an eligible professional (EP) or group practice under CMS guidelines for PQRS to report cross-cutting measures?

    a. telehealth visit
    b. acceptance of assignment
    c. surgical procedure code
    d. hospital privileges

**108.** When reviewing the credentials of a newly hired physician, the HIM director finds that complaints of negligence had been made against the physician at a previous place of employment, but no action had been taken against the physician. Which is the most appropriate response?

    a. Question the physician about the complaints before taking further action.
    b. Refer the information to the peer review committee/appropriate authority.
    c. Keep the information confidential since no action had been taken.
    d. Disqualify the physician from employment because of the complaints.

**109.** An external audit of coding practices should be conducted at least:

    a. monthly.
    b. yearly.
    c. every 2 years.
    d. every 5 years.

110. According to the history and physical notes, a 2-year-old child was brought to the emergency department, crying and pulling on his right ear. The mother stated that onset was earlier in the day. The left ear was clear but the right ear showed redness and bulging tympanic membrane but no perforation or drainage. The mother admitted to smoking "a few" cigarettes a day in the home environment. The child had been treated for bilateral otitis media 6 months previously. The physician listed the diagnoses as:

- Acute otitis media, right ear.
- Exposure to secondhand smoke.

**Which of the ICD-10-CM codes below are appropriate?**

| Diseases in the middle ear and mastoid (H65-H75) |
| --- |
| Use additional code to identify:<br>Z77.22 Exposure to environmental tobacco smoke<br>Z72.0 Tobacco use |
| H65 Nonsuppurative otitis media<br>H65 Acute serous otitis media<br>H65.00 unspecified ear<br>H65.01 right ear<br>H65.02 left ear<br>H65.03 bilateral<br>H65.04 recurrent, right ear<br>H65.05 recurrent. left ear<br>H65.06 recurrent, bilateral<br>H66 Suppurative and unspecified otitis media<br>H66.00 Acute suppurative otitis media without spontaneous rupture of the eardrum<br>H66.001 right ear<br>H66.002 left ear<br>H66.003 bilateral<br>H66.004 recurrent right ear<br>H66.005 recurrent left ear<br>H66.006 recurrent bilateral |

- a. H66.001, Z72.0
- b. H66.004, Z77.22
- c. H65.01, Z77.22
- d. H65.04, Z77.22

111. Following a 60-day hospitalization for complications related to diabetes and amputation of the right lower leg, the patient requested copies of the entire health record. Which of the following is *not* correct?

- a. The patient has a right to access the entire record.
- b. The hospital may charge a reasonable fee to cover costs.
- c. The hospital can withhold sensitive notes.
- d. The patient must provide the copies within 30 days.

**112. If an RHIT receives a subpoena duces tecum, the technician is being directed to:**

a. verify that records are authentic.
b. review records for fraudulent practices.
c. testify about patient care.
d. bring records (copies or originals).

**113. In preparation for an HHS Office of Civil Rights (OCR) HIPAA audit, an organization should begin by:**

a. completing a risk assessment.
b. requesting preliminary guidelines.
c. warning all staff members of the impending audit.
d. conducting staff training.

**114. Based on the General Equivalence Mapping below, what conclusion can be made about mapping the ICD-9-CM code 281.2, Folate deficiency anemia, to ICD-10-CM?**

| ICD-9-CM | Description | ICD-10-CM | Description | Approximate |
|----------|-------------|-----------|-------------|-------------|
| 281.2 | Folate deficiency anemia | D52.0 | Dietary folate deficiency anemia | 1 |
| 281.2 | Folate deficiency anemia | D52.1 | Drug-induced folate deficiency anemia | 1 |
| 281.2 | Folate deficiency anemia | D52.8 | Other folate deficiency anemias | 1 |
| 281.2 | Folate deficiency anemia | D52.9 | Folate deficiency anemia, unspecified | 1 |

a. 281.2 maps approximately to four ICD-10-CM codes.
b. 281.2 maps directly to an ICD-10-CM code.
c. 281.2 does not map to ICD-10-CM codes.
d. 281.2 maps directly to one ICD-10-CM and approximately to three ICD-10-CM codes.

**115. The HIM director is responsible for conducting an internal coding audit. The first step should be to:**

a. determine the scope of the audit.
b. identify those who will perform the audit.
c. gather reference materials needed for the audit.
d. identify items needed, such as charge tickets.

**116. When reviewing hospital statistics for hospital-acquired infections (HACs), the HIM director finds that the predicted number of surgical site infections (SSIs) for the hospital is 15, but 26 patients developed surgical site infections. This represents a standardized infection ratio (SIR) of:**

a. 3.90.
b. 0.57.
c. 17.3.
d. 1.73.

**117. Knowledge discovery in databases (KDD) is a method utilized to search databases in order to:**

    a. collect and summarize data.
    b. identify patterns and relationships.
    c. apply a standardized coding system
    d. translate analog data into digital.

**118. Which of the following healthcare providers is allowed to file a CMS claim for "incident to" services provide to a patient by auxiliary personnel?**

    a. the patient's physician.
    b. any physician certifying the services were provided.
    c. the physician providing direct supervision.
    d. any physician with knowledge about the services provided.

**119. Following FDA approval of an item and during the time when a new code is being considered for this item through the HCPCS review process, which type of HCPCS level II code should be utilized?**

    a. Permanent national codes
    b. Temporary codes
    c. Miscellaneous codes
    d. No codes can be utilized.

**120. A 70-year-old patient came to the emergency department for a right wrist injury and an x-ray showed a non-displaced Colles fracture. A short arm prefabricated splint was applied. How would the diagnosis, x-ray, splint, and splint application be coded for CMS billing?**

    a. ICD-10-CM for diagnosis, CPT for x-ray, CPT for splint application, and HCPCS level II L code for the splint.
    b. ICD-10-CM for diagnosis, CPT for x-ray, CPT for splint application, and CPT for splint.
    c. ICD-10-CM for diagnosis, HCPCS level II R code for x-ray, CPT for splint application, and CPT for splint.
    d. ICD-10-CM for diagnosis, CPT for x-ray, and HCPCS level II code L for splint (includes application).

**121. If a neoplasm is described with the term "adenoma" or "lipoma," which column in the ICD-10-CM Table of Neoplasms would the RHIT use to identify the correct code?**

    a. Malignant primary
    b. Malignant secondary
    c. Unspecified
    d. Benign

**122. A patient has a primary diagnosis of prostatic cancer (C61) but is admitted for radiation treatment (Z51.0) for metastasis to the bones (C79.51), and has also been receiving long-term treatment for diabetes mellitus, type 2, with polyneuropathy (E11.42). How would these diagnoses be sequenced (first to last)?**

    a. Z51.0, C79.51, C61, E11.42
    b. Z51.0, C61, C79.51, E11.42
    c. E11.42, Z51.0, C61, C79.51
    d. E11.42, C79.51, C61, Z51.0

**123. Which of the following NDCs is in the correct format for filing a CMS claim for a drug administered to a patient in an outpatient clinic?**

- a. 21695-0245-20
- b. 0069-5510-16
- c. 76237-134-30
- d. 17856-0079-1

**124. If a patient's diagnosis is "MRSA [methicillin-resistant *Staphylococcus aureus*] septicemia," which of the following is the most specific supporting documentation in the EHR?**

- a. Blood culture and sensitivities
- b. Chest x-ray
- c. Metabolic panel
- d. Complete blood cell count

**125. Which of the following is generally *not* part of the criteria for medical necessity?**

- a. Care is provided within clinically accepted medical practice standards.
- b. Care is appropriate to the patient's diagnosis, needs, and condition.
- c. Care is provided to restore health or prevent deterioration of health.
- d. Care is provided for maintenance or caregiver convenience.

**126. If the same information about a patient is entered into more than one table in a database, this is an example of:**

- a. data inconsistency.
- b. data redundancy.
- c. data replication.
- d. data disparity.

**127. Which of the following is a provision of a Voluntary Data Sharing Agreement (VDSA) with CMS?**

- a. Electronic exchange of health insurance benefit information
- b. Increased administrative costs
- c. Increased risk of repayment claims and penalties
- d. Electronic security system to protect information

**128. If, under HIPAA's Security Rule, a healthcare organization determines that an "addressable" implementation specification is not applicable or appropriate for the organization, the healthcare organization must:**

- a. Implement an alternate measure in place of the addressable measure.
- b. Document the decision and rationale and show how the standard is met.
- c. Implement the addressable implementation specification anyway.
- d. File an appeal requesting the organization be excused from implementation.

**129. Which of the TRICARE programs is an HMO style plan?**

- a. TRICARE Standard.
- b. TRICARE Extra.
- c. TRICARE Prime.
- d. TRICARE Guard and Reserve.

**130. If a database notes that a field is empty and displays an error message to remind the user to complete the field, this is an example of a(n):**

a. range check.
b. alphabetic check.
c. consistency check.
d. completeness check.

**131. A patient was hospitalized under Medicare 2 times in 1 year for extended periods of time because of complications associated with a BK amputation and sepsis. Sixty days separated the discharge from the first hospitalization to the admission for the second:**

    92 days.
    106 days.

**If the daily coinsurance per each lifetime reserve day is $644, for how much of the costs will the patient be financially responsible?**

a. None
b. $3,864
c. $5796
d. $11,592

**132. How much more in resources are generally required of a MS-DRG with a relative weight of 4.000 compared with a MS-DRG with a relative weight of 2.000?**

a. One-quarter as many
b. One-half as many
c. Twice as many
d. Four times as many

**133. If Hospital A and Hospital B both serve the same community, have 450 beds, discharge approximately the same number of patients, and have similar services, but Hospital A has a CMI of 1.57 and Hospital B has a CMI of 0.98, what is the most likely reason for the difference?**

a. Hospital A is carrying out unnecessary treatments.
b. Hospital B is not coding or capturing levels of severity adequately.
c. Hospital B has made an error in data used for CMI calculations.
d. Hospital A is a better hospital than Hospital B.

**134. Under APC guidelines, to qualify for outlier payments, the cost must exceed _____times the APC payment.**

a. 1.5
b. 2
c. 2.5
d. 3

**135. When calculating the CMI, the required data include:**

a. Wage index of each MS-DRG and the number of discharges in the MS-DRG
b. Wage index of each MS-DRG and the number of admissions in the MS-DRG
c. Relative weight of each MS-DRG and the number of admissions in the MS-DRG
d. Relative weight of each MS-DRG and number of discharges in the MS-DRG

**136. According to the A/R report, the greatest percentage of aged bills occurs in which time period?**

| Patient A/R Report | | | Days outstanding | | | | | |
| ID | Name | Current | 31-60 | 91-120 | 121-150 | 151-180 | 180+ | Total |
| --- | --- | --- | --- | --- | --- | --- | --- | --- |
| 001 | Doe, J | | | | | | 28.56 | 28.56 |
| 708 | Jones, M | | 42.88 | | | 663.00 | | 705.88 |
| 889 | Lee, J | 178.00 | 217.00 | | 128.78 | | | 523.78 |
| 997 | Jong, M | | | 2850.00 | | 526.42 | | 3376.42 |
| 662 | Brown, A | | | 1066.10 | | | 2896.00 | 3962.10 |
| Totals: | | 178.00 | 259.88 | 3916.10 | 128.78 | 1189.42 | 2924.56 | 8596.74 |

   a. 31-60
   b. 91-120
   c. 151-180
   d. 180+

**137. According to the SNF Consolidated Billing (CB) requirement, which of the following must be included on the Part A bill for Medicare-covered services?**
   a. Only PT, OT, and SLP services provided directly by the SNF.
   b. Services of qualified psychologists.
   c. Hospice care for end-of-life management for a patient.
   d. All PT, OT, and SLP services received by the patient.

**138. After a claim is entered into a payer's system, which action occurs next?**
   a. A payer data file is established.
   b. Claim information is reviewed against the payer's data file.
   c. Computerized edits are conducted to assess services and coding.
   d. Allowable charges are determined and payment sent.

**139. The three types of edits that are carried out by the Medicare Code Editor (MCE) are:**
   a. inpatient coding, coverage, and inpatient clinical.
   b. inpatient coding, claims, and coverage.
   c. inpatient coding, claims, and inpatient clinical.
   d. claims, coverage, and clinical.

**140. In the Medicare appeals process, which of the following is the first level of appeals?**
   a. Reconsideration
   b. Hearing
   c. Redetermination
   d. Review

**141. According to the federal False Claims Act, if a provider bills Medicare $250.00 for services that were not provided to the patient and later submits another claim for $125 for services not provided, how much would the fine be if the provider were found guilty of filing fraudulent claims?**
   a. $375
   b. $10,375
   c. $11,125
   d. $21,125

**142.** If a healthcare organization shows a profit of $120,000 on $2 million dollars in revenue, the organization's profit margin is:

    a. 2%
    b. 4%
    c. 6%
    d. 8%

**143.** The HIM director created a chart to show the number of complaints received in 1-week period about the EHR system. Based on these results, what action is most indicated?

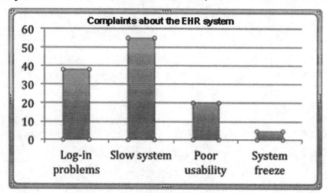

    a. Conduct staff training regarding use of the EHR system.
    b. Conduct further surveys to gain more definitive results.
    c. Conduct system testing to identify problems and improve performance.
    d. Conduct usability testing to determine training needs.

**144.** In the conversion from paper records to the EHR, the HIM department must make a decision about back-scanning. Back-scanning refers to scanning:

    a. paper records already in existence.
    b. planned for a future time.
    c. claim-supporting documents only.
    d. discharge summaries only of paper records.

**145.** The best method of establishing productivity goals for coding professionals is to:

    a. calculate goals based on needs, number of staff, and number of hours.
    b. measure actual production over a specified period of time.
    c. survey staff about what they consider reasonable goals.
    d. estimate based on past experience and observation.

**146.** As part of the clinical documentation management program (CDMP) to improve documentation of medical necessity and decrease coding errors at a large teaching hospital, coders have been assigned in teams to code for specialty units, such as oncology and cardiac care. The next step should be to:

    a. assign team leaders.
    b. set productivity goals.
    c. provide incentive pay for improved performance.
    d. provide specialty unit-specific training.

**147.** If using CPT code 20680 (removal of implant, deep) for a hardware removal procedure after a physician removed a plate and 3 screws for an orthopedic injury because of a metal sensitivity reaction, how many times should the code be entered on the claim form?

a. one time
b. two times
c. three times
d. four times

**148.** What is the recommended time period that a healthcare facility should retain the register of surgical procedures?

a. 1 year
b. 5 years
c. 10 years
d. Permanently

**149.** Which healthcare provider is *not* able to legally diagnose and write medical orders?

a. Nurse Practitioner (NP)
b. Physician Assistant (PA)
c. Registered nurse (RN)
d. Physician (MD)

**150.** If the master patient index (MPI) includes a *Soundex* field, how would the name "Parker" be coded?

| Letter | Code | Letter | Code |
|---|---|---|---|
| B, F, P, V | 1 | M, N | 5 |
| C, G, J, K, Q, S, X, Z | 2 | R | 6 |
| D, T | 3 | A, E, I, O, W, Y | No code |
| L | 4 | If less than 3 digits long | Add 0 |

a. 1626
b. P626
c. P6-6
d. 16-6

**151.** A healthcare provider's fee is $180, but the provider has agreed to a write-down adjustment of $40 from the insurance company. However, the insurance company only directly pays 75% and the patient pays 25% as a copayment. How much is the insurance company's actual reimbursement?

a. $140
b. $115
c. $105
d. $75

**152.** A "bill-hold period" is used by HIM to ensure that:

a. all charges are posted on the claim.
b. copies of the bills are retained for a specified time period.
c. claims are sent out in batches.
d. payers have adequate time to make payment.

**153. What is the purpose of grouper software?**

    a. Classify patients into the correct MS-DRG.
    b. Facilitate data mining for clinical research.
    c. Group patients according to admitting diagnosis.
    d. Group patients according to demographic information.

**154. When a claim is submitted to CMS, the factors that affect the MS-DRG reimbursement are:**

    a. hospital IPPS rate and LOS.
    b. relative weight and hospital IPPS rate.
    c. relative weight and LOS.
    d. relative weight only.

**155. In a transaction-processing system, a detailed report about admissions would be classified as a(n):**

    a. transaction.
    b. product.
    c. input.
    d. output.

**156. For the Medicare fee schedule that lists allowable charges for physicians under Medicare B, the factors that are utilized when calculating relative value units (RVUs) and geographic practice cost indices (GPCIs) include all of the following *except*:**

    a. physician work.
    b. practice expense.
    c. specialty licensure.
    d. malpractice costs.

**157. In the OPPS, what does an "N" status indicator mean?**

    a. No APC rate exists for this service.
    b. Service will receive partial payment.
    c. Service will be discounted.
    d. Service/item is packaged into the APC rate.

**158. If further information is needed to complete coding of a patient's record and the physician must be queried, which of the following is likely the most efficient method?**

    a. telephone call
    b. query form
    c. text message
    d. personal interview

159. With medical and surgical procedures in ICD-10-PCS, which meanings are missing in the chart demonstrating the seven characters utilized for coding?

| 1 | 2 | 3 | 4 | 5 | 6 | 7 |
|---|---|---|---|---|---|---|
| Section | Body system | Root operation | | | Device | Qualifier |

    a. (4) Body part, (5) Approach
    b. (4) Approach, (5) Body part
    c. (4) Body part, (5) Severity
    d. (4) Approach, (5) Severity

160. If a primary care physician (PCP) in an HMO receives payment based on *capitation*, this means that:

    a. there is a cap on the amount of fees the PCP can charge.
    b. the PCP is paid a flat fee for each patient visit.
    c. the PCP is paid a flat fee for each of his/her patients enrolled in the HMO.
    d. the PCP receives a specific monthly fee regardless of the number of his/her patients.

161. If two hospitals each have the same number of licensed beds but the first hospital (X) has an ALOS of 3 and discharges 30,000 patients per year and the second hospital (Y) has an ALOS of 6 and discharges 15,000 per year, which hospital has the greater capacity?

    a. Capacity is equal.
    b. Data are insufficient.
    c. Hospital Y
    d. Hospital X

162. As part of utilization management, intensity-of-service screening and severity of illness (ISSI) criteria are used to:

    a. determine whether a patient needs continued inpatient care.
    b. determine if proposed inpatient care is a medical necessity.
    c. determine whether a patient needs inpatient care based on physical impairment.
    d. determine whether a patient requires inpatient or outpatient care.

163. Serious medical errors occurred in an acute care facility because physicians and nursing staff persistently used workarounds to the EHR, such as copying and pasting information and writing information and orders on paper for later entry. When considering steps to remedy the situation, the HIM director understands that the most common reason for workarounds is:

    a. staff resistance to technology.
    b. EHR design incompatible with work processes.
    c. inadequate staff training.
    d. inadequate staffing and overwork.

164. When conducting testing on health information technology projects in the health information management department, testing should be done in which of the following orders?

    a. (1) system, (2) integration, (3) unit, (4) usability
    b. (1) unit, (2) integration, (3) system, (4) usability
    c. (1) system, (2) unit, (3) usability, (4) integration
    d. (1) unit, (2) system, (3) integration, (4) usability

**165. Which data set is designed to gather data about Medicare patients who are under the care of a home health agency?**

    a.  OASIS-CI

    b.  MDS

    c.  UCDS

    d.  DEEDS

# Answer Key and Explanations

**1. D:** If a hospital has a base MS-DRG of $5040.00 and the following adjustments are made

Value based purchasing (VBP): (-$5.06)

Disproportionate share hospital (DSH): +$128.56

Indirect medical education (IME): +$486.22

Readmission adjustment: (-$1.08)

So, the new base operating MS-DRG (subject to case mix) is $5648.64.

Calculations:

$$\$5040 - 5.06 + 128.56 + 486.22 - 1.08 = \$5648.64$$

**2. B:** The RUG-IV group classification system is used in the SNF PPS. Patients are classified into RUGs based on acuity with patients requiring heavy care paid for at a higher reimbursement rate than those requiring lighter care. RUG-IV calculations take into consideration late-loss ADL score and total therapy minutes. Late-loss ADL's are heavily weighted and include those activities that patients often are able to retain the longest: bed mobility, toilet use, transfer, and eating.

**3. C:** A HIPAA-covered entity that experiences a security breach that resulted in unauthorized access of PHI of 650 (more than 500) individuals must not only notify the individuals involved within 60 days but must also notify HHS and the local news media within 60 days. The local news media must be notified because it is often not possible to notify each individual because of change of address or insufficient information. The organization must document the breach on a data security breach log and submit this log to HHS on an annual basis.

**4. C:** RxNorm allows health organizations and pharmacies to communicate drug-related information efficiently. RxNorm comprises a naming system for drugs (generic and branded) and tools that allows interoperability. Drugs are provided unique identifiers so that information about drugs can be provided consistently across different systems. Dietary supplements, bulk powders, contrast media, and durable medical equipment are not included in RxNorm. RxNorm collects data for 14 different terminologies.

**5. A:** While a full discharge summary is necessary for most admissions, if the stay is uncomplicated and lasts for fewer than 48 hours, a discharge note may be acceptable. Typically, if a patient is admitted for normal childbirth and stays less than 48 hours, only the discharge note is needed. However, it is important to determine the policy of each institution as policies may vary. A discharge summary provides a complete overview of the patient's encounter with medical care, transmitting information needed by the patient's attending physician or other healthcare providers to ensure continuity of care.

**6. D:** In addition to the CDT (Current Dental Terminology) code for removal of a tooth, the other information that is required is the tooth number (1 to 32). CDT comprises 12 service codes (diagnostic, preventive, restorative, endodontics, periodontics, prosthodontics-removable, maxillofacial prosthetics, implant services, prosthodontics-fixed, oral and maxillofacial surgery,

33

orthodontics, and adjunctive general services). Each category has a code series and a number of subcategories that vary according to the category.

**7. B:** If a patient is admitted primarily for management of pain caused by a malignancy (G89.3), the pain control is listed as the principle diagnosis, followed by the malignancy causing the pain (C25.0), the malignant neoplasm of the head of the pancreas. (Admissions for therapy also list the therapy code before the malignancy code.) Other diagnoses, such as the anemia, follow. Anemia is not the purpose for this admission. Coding sequence:

G89.3, C25.0, and D64.81.

**8. C:** The most important accrediting agency for acute care and ambulatory care is the Joint Commission (TJC), which conducts accreditation surveys on a minimum cycle of every 3 years, although some changes in standards may occur each year, so organizations must keep current with changes and implement measures to ensure compliance with all standards. The Joint Commission also sets standards and accredits long-term care facilities, rehabilitation centers, hospices, and home health agencies.

**9. B:** Medicare will waive an organization's need for a compliance audit if it is appropriately accredited, such as by the Joint Commission, by granting it deemed status. This means that the accreditation ensures that the CMS conditions of participation (COP) have been adequately met, and the organization can receive reimbursement for care provided. The deemed organization meets certification requirements for CMS and does not, therefore, need to undergo the compliance audit.

**10. A:** When a patient has a gallbladder surgically removed and the specimen is examined in the laboratory and a report is generated that describes the gross appearance as well as the microscopic findings, this report is referred to as a pathology report. A typical pathology report would include the type of specimen, the size, shape, and general gross appearance (macroscopic), as well as an explanation of microscopic findings, such as cell type and whether a specimen is malignant or benign. Last, a diagnosis, based on the specimen, is provided.

**11. C:** If a hospital has 200 licensed beds available and 150 of those beds are occupied with patients, the current occupancy rate is 75%, the percentage of beds in use in a designated period. To calculate, the number of days the beds are occupied is divided by the total number of beds available. Occupancy rates are usually based on licensed beds, but some facilities may calculate using bed count, especially if some parts of the facility are closed to patients so that the beds are not available. However, using the number of licensed beds gives a more stable number.

**12. C:** Under the IRF PPS, if a patient is discharged from a rehabilitation facility on July 16, the date by which the data transmission of the discharge patient assessment instrument (PAI) to CMS is considered late is August 12. The data must be transmitted no later than 27 calendar days after the patient is discharged. The PAI must be completed within 4 days of discharge (by July 20) and encoded within an additional 6 days (by July 26). The discharge PAI is transmitted electronically to the CMS.

**13. A:** While the 12N to 7PM time period started out with the longest wait time and this persisted for 4 months, this time period has the greatest overall improvement, decreasing from a wait time of 58 minutes in January to a wait time of 32 minutes in June. The 7AM to 12N time period, however, showed the smallest decrease of any time period as its lowest wait time (38) was only 6 minutes lower than the January wait time (44), so this time period would likely benefit the most from additional staffing.

**14. B:** If a staff member of a healthcare facility has authorized access to ePHI but has given 2 weeks' notice of intent to resign, the procedure that must be implemented when the person resigns is the termination procedure. Access privileges must be immediately removed on the day the person leaves employment so that the person cannot access any data. Termination procedures must be documented with steps clearly outlined so that the procedures can be applied with equity.

**15. C:** If a hospital with 300 licensed and available beds has an average length of stay (ALOS) of 5 days, the hospital could serve 1800 patients in a 30-day period. Calculation:

$$[\text{Number of beds}] \times [\text{number of days}] \div [\text{ALOS}]$$

$$300 \times 30 = 9000 \text{ total bed days available}$$

$$\text{ALOS} = 5$$

$$9000 \div 5 = 1800 \text{ patients}$$

The lower the ALOS, the more patients a hospital is able to serve.

**16. A:** The standard format that is used by hospitals and other institutional providers to transmit health claims electronically to CMS is 837I. Almost all hospitals now submit claims electronically, as mandated by HIPAA's Administrative Simplification Compliance Act (ASCA). The standard 837I replaces UB-04 (CMS-1450), which was used for paper billing and may still be used for facilities with a waiver. Physicians use 837P to submit claims instead of the CMS-1500 paper billing form.

**17. D:** Patients in acute care facilities, often referred to as hospitals, usually do not stay more than 30 days maximum because those in need of care longer than 30 days are most often transferred to other facilities, such as subacute care facilities, rehabilitation centers, and long-term care facilities, such as nursing homes, skilled nursing facilities, and residential care facilities. Patients may also be sent home under the care of a home health agency.

**18. B:** The department in an acute care facility that is considered an outpatient department rather than inpatient is the emergency department (ED). The ED is an outpatient department because patients are not admitted formally to the acute care facility and stay for a limited period of time. Other outpatient departments may include laboratory and radiology services as well as ambulatory surgery centers where people have a surgical procedure and are generally discharged the same day.

**19. C:** If a patient is admitted to an acute care facility at 11:50 PM on May 2 and discharged at 7 AM on May 6, the LOS is 4 days. To calculate the LOS, count the first day as the date of admission, regardless of the hour, and then count each day up to the date of discharge. The date of discharge is not counted. Thus, the patient was present on the 2nd, 3rd, 4th, and 5th (four days), and then discharged on the 6th.

**20. A:** HL7 refers to Health Level Seven. HL7 is an organization that develops international standards used in the sharing, retrieval, exchange, and integration of electronic health information. HL7 is accredited by the American National Standards Institute (ANSI). There are seven categories of standards: primary, foundational, clinical and administrative domains, EHR profiles, implementation guides, rule and references, and education and awareness.

**21. D:** The Health Insurance Portability and Accountability Act (HIPAA) was passed by Congress in 1996. HIPAA has had a profound effect on health information management because it mandates that the privacy of patient records be protected and establishes specific standards to be used for data codes and sets. Additionally, HIPAA requires that security provisions be taken for patient records that are stored electronically to prevent unauthorized access to electronic protected health information (ePHI).

**22. B:** Authorizations are used to indicate a patient's permission to disclose PHI, such as when sending health records to an employer or to a different physician. While the forms may vary in appearance, HIPAA regulations require that they contain some specific elements. The consent for treatment is not among these elements. Elements include the date the form was signed, the expiration date, the name of the person/entity to whom information will be disclosed, the information that may be disclosed, and the purpose.

**23. A:** In table 1 (the parent table) a relational database, Emp_No is the primary key because it is a unique identifier and no other employee can have that number. The primary key may be in one column or a combination of columns. The foreign key Emp_No in table 2 (the child table) links the two tables by referring to the primary key of table 1. Any data in the foreign key column should have corresponding value in the table to which it is linked.

**24. D:** The Security Rule of HIPAA applies to ePHI (whether created, received, stored, or transmitted) only, while the Privacy Rule applies to all forms of PHI (paper, oral, electronic). The Security Rule includes comprehensive security requirements in order to safeguard ePHI. These requirements are more stringent than for other forms of PHI. The Security Rule is enforced by CMS while the Privacy Rule is enforced by the Office of Civil Rights (OCR).

**25. C:** If the HIM department plans user acceptance testing (UAT) to determine if the end users are willing and able to use new equipment and applications as intended, the first step to analyzing end-user acceptance is to determine the basic system and organization requirements so that the test can be designed about those requirements. The scenarios for end-user acceptance should be identified and the severity levels of the testing plan described. Test cases and the testing plan should be designed with the skills of the end users in mind.

**26. D:** A group of 8 bits makes one byte, a basic computing unit. In an 8-bit byte, the beginning value of bit 1 is 1, but each succeeding bit doubles in value (2, 4, 8, 16, 32, 64, and 128). If all of the values are activated and are added together, the maximum value of a byte in terms of bits is 256 bits. The bit is the smallest information unit. The computer utilizes this system for the binary (two part) number system.

**27. B:** In a relational database, the data are separated into defined logical groups by fields, which can be alphanumeric (text), numeric, or dates, and may be whole numbers or decimals. The field is the second level of a database with characters composing the first level. Characters are the smallest unit of text data as defined by the ASCII table. The third level is the record, which comprises a group of fields about a specific topic or thing. Records can then be grouped into tables.

**28. A:** If a healthcare organization has no formal policy regarding computer/Internet use but the administration asks the HIM department to monitor employee emails and Internet use, the appropriate response is that the administration must first establish written policies regarding computer/Internet use in order to avoid violating employee's right to privacy. Restrictions on use in the workplace must be clearly outlined, including any disciplinary action that may be taken for violations. The policy should also clearly state the type of monitoring that will occur.

**29. B:** If an acute care hospital invested in new diagnostic equipment at a cost of $520,000 and showed a benefit of $825,000 at the end of the year, the return on investment (ROI) (rounded to the nearest whole number) is 59%. ROI formula:

$$\text{ROI(expressed in percentage)} = \frac{\text{Total benefits} - \text{total costs}}{\text{total costs}} \times 100$$
$$= \frac{825,000 - 520,000}{520,000} \times 100$$
$$= \frac{305,000}{520,000} \times 100$$
$$= 0.586 \times 100$$
$$= 59\%$$

**30. C:** When a patient is admitted to a hospital, the registration clerk should check the master patient index (MPI) to ensure that a duplicate record is not created for a patient who is already registered in the system. The MPI is a secondary health record that is usually computerized and that contains key identifying information, such as name, birthdate, and ID number or social security number, for patients registered anywhere in the system. Even though a new health record may be created with each admission, the same key identifying information will be in each record.

**31. A:** According to the American Health Information Management Association's (AHIMA's) minimum retention schedule, diagnostic images, such as x-rays, should be retained for 5 years. Paper records are generally shredded and/or incinerated. The reality is that electronic records are often stored for longer periods, even permanently, because of ease of storage, low storage cost, and presence of electronic backups of data. However, when electronic storage equipment is disposed of, the PHI must be permanently removed from the equipment being disposed of so that the data cannot be accessed.

**32. B:** In order to determine how may FTE coders are needed to meet additional coding needs, the total number of items in each category is divided by the current productivity rate per hour:

$$500/2.5 = 200$$
$$420/3.5 = 120$$
$$840/7 = 120$$
$$800/10 = 80$$

$$200 + 120 + 120 + 80 = 520 \text{ total hours}$$
$$(520 \text{ hours})/(40 \text{ hours}) = 13 \text{ FTE coders}$$

**33. C:** An example of a primary purpose for an electronic health record is patient care management. Primary purposes are associated with direct care of the patient and documenting encounters between the patient and healthcare providers. Other primary purposes include delivering patient care, providing patient care support processes, determining reimbursement for care, and allowing the patient to engage in self-management through access to the health record. Secondary purposes are not associated with direct care and may include such things as providing evidence in litigation, engaging in clinical research, and allocating resources.

**34. D:** If a physician completed history and physical exam documentation 3 to 5 days after the physician actually conducted the history and physical examinations for 20 patients, the quality characteristic of data quality management that has been violated is data currency. For data to have currency, it must be up-to-date and documented or recorded at the time the history and physical examinations were carried out or immediately after. Attempting to recall details for numerous patients after an elapsed time period may result in inaccuracy of data.

**35. A:** The process through which data are archived is referred to as data warehousing. Data warehouses are centralized repositories of information collected from a variety of sources and stored for future use. Data warehouses may be mined for data when collecting aggregate data for research purposes or for reports. Data may be warehoused to meet the minimum retention time, such as 5 years for images (x-rays, CTs, MRIs). AHIMA's data quality management is based on the 4 domains of data warehousing, data applications, data collection, and data analysis.

**36. C:** If paper health records are filed using terminal digit filing and a patient's health record is numbered 44-62-10, the chart will be filed in section 10 as the last digits are the primary set of numbers referred to for filing purposes, and the middle set (62) is the secondary set, indicating the correct subsection in section 10. The chart will be placed between charts 43 and 45 in subsection 62 in section 10. Other filing methods include straight numeric filing, alphanumeric filing (initials of patient precede number), and middle digit filing.

**37. D:** The Joint Commission accredits a wide range of healthcare facilities and organizations, including acute care hospitals, children's hospitals, psychiatric institutions, rehabilitation centers, clinical laboratories, long-term care facilities, and home health agencies. National Committee for Quality assurance (NCQA) accredits managed care organizations as well as wellness and health promotion and managed behavioral health organizations. Accreditation Association for Ambulatory Health Care (AAAHC) accredits ambulatory care facilities, office-based surgery centers, and managed care organizations. Commission on Accreditation of Rehabilitation Facilities (CARF) accredits rehabilitation programs.

**38. B:** In a paper record filing system, an outguide is used to track files that have been checked out. The outguide is usually a colored plastic folder that is inserted into the space where the record had been. The outguide has a pocket to contain documents that arrive after the record has been removed and must be included in the record as well as a pocket to contain information about who checked out the record and when so that the record can be located.

**39. C:** Security standards include:

Technical safeguards: Encrypting and decrypting data while it is being stored or transmitted from one place to another. Utilization of authentication controls to ensure that those accessing data are authorized to do so.

Administrative safeguards: Ensuring that requirements for training are met and delegating responsibility for security.

Physical safeguards: Restricting access to ePHI and retaining computer backups offsite. Protecting equipment, data, and software from threats, intrusions, and hazards.

**40. A:**

**Clinic_Patients**

| Pat_ID | Last_Name | First_Name | Clinic | Ad_Date |
|--------|-----------|------------|----------|------------|
| 001 | Evans | Maria | WellBaby | 01/06/2016 |
| 002 | Locke | James | HIV_AIDS | 12/03/2015 |

If using SQL to query a relational database with the headings as in the table above, the correct query for a list of patient IDs and patient names for patients who attended the Well-Baby clinic only is:

SELECT Pat_ID, Last_Name, First_Name, Clinic FROM Clinic_Patients

WHERE Clinic = 'WellBaby'

**41. D:** If a physician uses another staff person's password to access data about a patient, this type of patient data misuse is an example of unauthorized access, even if the patient is under the care of the physician. The facility should have a way for the physician to obtain a lost or forgotten password. Since passwords are coded to specific individuals, it will appear in the record that the password owner accessed the record rather than the physician.

**42. B:** The PHR (personal health record) differs from the EHR in that the PHR is controlled by the individual. PHRs vary considerably, but in many cases contain not only information entered by the individual but also information from all healthcare providers. The PHR is a secure file, and only authorized access through appropriate user names and passwords is allowed, although it can be easily accessed from any location. The information usually covers a patient's lifetime rather than just the current illness or healthcare encounter.

**43. A:** There would be cost benefit of $29,600. The current annual overtime costs are:

$$\$125 \times 40 = \$5000 \times 12 \text{ months} = \$60,000$$

The HIM department proposes reducing these costs to 10 hours monthly:

$$\$125 \times 10 = \$1250 \times 12 \text{ months} = \$15,000$$

$$\$60,000 - \$15,000 = \$45,000 \text{ proposed reduction in costs.}$$

Cost include:

$$(\text{supplies}) + (\text{instructor}) + (6 \text{ staff}) = \$400 + \$3000 + \$12,000 = \$15,400$$

Cost benefit:

$$\$45,000 - \$15,400 = \$29,600$$

**44. C:** If the HIM department must purchase or lease new hardware to replace an outdated system and has identified four potential vendors, the next step in the vendor selection process is to send an RFI (request for information) to each company, which should provide general information that can be used to further screen the companies and narrow the field. Then, a request for proposal (RFP) is sent to the remaining potential vendors. At this point, vendors are evaluated and the top candidates selected before contract negotiations begin.

**45. D:** When conducting trending analysis of data in a run chart, a *run* occurs with $\geq 7$ data consecutive data points all above or all below the median. A *trend* occurs with $\geq 7$ consecutive data points in either ascending or descending order with $\geq 21$ total data points or $\geq 6$ with fewer than 21 total data points. A *cycle* occurs with up and down variation forming a sawtooth pattern with 14 successive data points. An *astronomical value* occurs with data point unrelated to other points (indicating a sentinel event).

**46. A:** If the laboratory in an acute hospital has begun sending automated alerts by instant messaging to physicians for all abnormal lab results rather than telephoning to try to improve response rate, but studies show that many alerts are ignored and response time has only slightly improved, the best method to improve response time is likely to reset parameters for alerts for all tests. Slight abnormalities in laboratory studies are common but often not clinically significant, and when physicians are inundated with unnecessary alerts, they tend to ignore them.

**47. C:** If, prior to upgrading to a new EHR system, the HIM department conducts workplace analysis to ensure the EHR integrates well into the clinical workflow, the initial step should be to assess the current status. This includes reviewing the document management system and processes involved as well as security provisions. The movement of documents, materials, data, and people (staff, patients, physicians) through a system should be assessed.

**48. D:** If an acute care hospital has instituted barcodes on patient ID bracelets and medications in order to decrease medicine errors in order to comply with National Patient Safety Goals, but nurses are copying the barcodes and placing them on the medicine cart for scanning so that they can prepare a number of different medicines at one time to deliver later to patients, this practice is never acceptable as ID is not at the point of care. The nurse could easily deliver the wrong medication to a patient.

**49. B:** To ensure that a hospital's EHR aligns with the CMS EHR Incentive Program, it is necessary to be 100% compliant with CMS required criteria to demonstrate Meaningful Use. The hospital acquires the certification ID by verifying that the EHR technology in use is on the Certified Health IT Product List. An automated guide to determine eligibility is available on the website of the Office of the National Coordinator for Health Information Technology (ONC).

**50. A:** Although the audit trail can be used for other purposes, such as identifying problems in the system and monitoring PHI imported from other systems, the primary purpose of reviewing the audit trails of an EHR is to determine if the EHR has undergone unauthorized access. The audit trail should show who has accessed an EHR and when, as well as any operations that were performed, such as downloading information or images.

**51. C:** The purpose of the compliance plans established by the Office of the Inspector General (OIG) is to ensure that organizations bill for services properly, including the avoidance of overcharging. If an organization routinely miscodes, resulting in overpayment, this can result in prosecution as an act of fraud. Therefore, internal controls to ensure that coding for billing purposes is done accurately are essential. Organizations should maintain written standards of conduct and should have compliance officers.

**52. B:** If a patient was admitted to the hospital for occlusion of the right femoral artery and underwent an open surgical procedure in which the right femoral artery was dilated with a drug-coated balloon and a drug-eluting stent placed in the lumen of the artery, the correct ICD-10-PCS code is "047K041 Dilation of right femoral artery with drug-eluting intraluminal device using drug-coated balloon, open approach." Nine procedure codes are associated with dilation of the right femoral artery.

**53. D:** In order to avoid medical records being classified as delinquent following discharge of patients from the hospital, records must be completed, including inclusion of the final diagnosis, within 30 days. For this reason, early review of the records should be carried out so that omissions in the records can be remedied prior to the end of the 30-day period. For accreditation by the Joint Commission, hospitals must audit delinquency rates at least every 3 months.

**54. A:** The ICD-10-CM that is non-covered by Medicare for all lab national coverage determinations (NCDs) is "Z00.01 Encounter for general adult medical examination with abnormal findings," as this indicates a screening test. Screening tests are generally non-covered unless coverage is specified by statute; however, if the screening results in an abnormal finding, as with Z00.01, then Z00.01 is the first line code, but a second code should be applied that accounts for the abnormal finding.

**55. B:** If creating a data dictionary to correspond to a patient information table with ID #, last name, first name, gender, and birthdate, the data dictionary would contain the field name, data length (maximum length of data that a field can accept), type of data (integer, alpha, double, date, long integer), and order of fields (according to listing). The data dictionary:

| Field Name | Length | Data type |
|---|---|---|
| ID # | 5 | Long integer |
| Last_Name | 24 | Alpha |
| First_Name | 22 | Alpha |
| Gender | 5 | Alpha |
| Birthdate | 10 | Date |

**56. A:** If the HIM director is planning to make changes in order to increase efficiency and wants to begin by carrying out a gap analysis, the first step in gap analysis is to identify best practices, which should represent the end target. Then, the next step is to assess how current practices diverge from the best practice. This helps to determine the gaps that exist. In addition, barriers to implementation of best practices should be identified. Barriers may include such things as lack of resources or lack of administrative support.

**57. B:** In a relational database, the three types of possible anomalies include:

Update: Redundancies occur in the data, so updates must be done more than once to cover all redundancies or the data error will not be corrected.

Insertion: Data cannot be added to a database because of the absence of other necessary data.

Deletion: Data are unintentionally lost when other data are deleted.

**58. C:** If two computers and a server were stolen because the door to the room with the equipment was left ajar, the type of security measure that is insufficient is physical safeguards. Equipment should be maintained behind locked doors, and the doors should close completely after opening. Alarms should sound if the door does not latch properly. Management practices include policies regarding privacy, confidentiality, and security. Technical measures include those that are included as part of software, such as the requirement for passwords.

**59. C:** A "warm" site with patient data should be located at least 50 miles away from a healthcare organization and at least 20 miles away from a coast. The distance should be great enough that the data are likely to be secure in the event of a natural disaster, such as a hurricane or flood hitting the healthcare organization, but close enough that it can be accessed and activated within 8 hours. This backup system should be able to run the EHR.

**60. B:** The type of incident that would usually result in the involvement of a law enforcement agency is if an employee is suspected of identity theft. Identity theft is an illegal act, but the crime is classified by states differently, ranging from misdemeanor to felony. Penalties may range from fines to imprisonment, and many states require complete restitution. In some states, identity thefts against older individuals carry an added penalty.

**61. A:** If, prior to the installation of a new computer system, the HIM department conducts volume testing, the purpose is to determine the upper limits at which the computer system can function adequately. The testing should be carried out so that it mimics peak use times as well as low volume times. The testing attempts to determine if there is a point at which system errors occur. Testing, both static and dynamic, should be done at a safe working load (SWL) and a higher than SWL.

**62. B:** When training new staff members in the HIM department about data flow within a healthcare organization, the best method is likely to provide a data-flow diagram that outlines in detail the ways in which data flows into a system and from process to process. The data flow diagram uses standardized symbols including the square (external entity/source of data or data destinations), rounded rectangles (process used to input or output data), arrow (direction of flow), and three-sided open triangle (data storage).

**63. D:** While there is a wide range of completion of records according to the clinical pertinence review, the data are insufficient to make accurate determinations about where review of procedures is most needed. There is no indication about the size (bed counts) of the departments or the numbers of physicians in each department. A further step may be to pull 10% of the records for each physician in the ONC department to determine if the rates are consistent with the department percentage or if one or more physicians have very low completion rates that are skewing the data.

**64. D:** If the HIM department is assisting in the development of a mobile device policy, insurance policy against loss is not a critical measure to include in the policy; however, the device should have remote disabling/wiping installed in the event that a device is lost. The Virtual Private Network (VPN) allows data to be transmitted securely from unsecured environments, such as a public Wi-Fi access points. Security and privacy training should be provided for all those using mobile device for transmission of health information.

**65. C:** If the County Hospital administration is considering transitioning to cloud storage and has asked the HIM department to assess vendors and gather information, the most important initial issue to consider is compliance with regulations. Data security is primary, so the vendor should verify that a company meets HIPAA requirements and complies with the Code of Federal Regulation, Title 21, Part 11, which outlines regulations about electronic records and signatures. Other issues to consider include initial and ongoing costs, vendor reputation, and interoperability.

**66. D:** If an audit of narcotic prescriptions in the emergency department shows that one physician has ordered 4 times more narcotics than any other physician in the department over a 1-month period with multiple prescriptions to some individuals, the most appropriate action is to alert the administration. Because the rate of prescriptions is so out of step with others, the likelihood exists that the physician is supplying drugs that are not necessary for medical health reasons.

**67. B:** HCPCS level II E codes are used when filing a Medicare claim for durable medical equipment, such as a bedside commode. D codes are used for dental procedures and include the CDT code set copyrighted by the American Dental Association (ADA). L codes are used for orthotic and prosthetic procedures and devices, such as orthopedic shoes. P codes are used for pathology and laboratory services.

**68. C:** As part of the review process for short-stay (fewer than 2 midnights) inpatients, the Quality Improvement Organization (QIO) acting for CMS will pull 20 short-stay inpatient records from small hospitals and 50 from large hospitals to determine medical necessity. The QIO will assess the

42

records to determine if the physician had a reasonable expectation that the hospitalization would exceed 2 midnights or the patient's condition, needs, or risk factors warranted inpatient hospitalization. Claim denials will be referred to the Medicare Administrative Contractors (MACS) for payment adjustment.

**69. A:** Under ICD-10-CM, unspecified codes are used when sufficient information about the condition is not yet available. For example, if a patient has otitis media, suppurative, in the right ear but the causative organism has not been identified, the diagnosis would be coded as H66.41, Suppurative otitis media, unspecified, right ear. The coder should be careful not to choose a code based on supposition about the probable diagnosis as the diagnosis must be supported by documentation in the patient's record.

**70. C:** DEEDS (Data Elements for Emergency Departments) is a data set published by the CDC in order to collect uniform data from emergency departments in hospitals, although participation is voluntary. The data set has 8 sections and includes data about patient ID, facility and practitioner ID, payment, arrival and first assessment, history and physical examination, procedures and results, medications, disposition and diagnosis. The data are utilized for public health surveillance and risk assessments, as well as research, training, and education.

**71. D:** When reporting other diagnoses or conditions beyond the primary diagnosis for UHDDS (Uniform Hospital Discharge Data Set), only other diagnoses or conditions associated with the current health services should be reported. Diagnoses should be ordered with the most severe listed first. Chronic conditions, such as hypertension or rheumatoid arthritis, should be reported because ongoing care is expected for chronic disorders. Previous diagnoses not associated with current medical services should not be reported.

**72. C:** The part of Medicare coverage that includes Medicare Advantage Plans is Part C. Medicare Advantage Plans are approved by Medicare but are under the auspices of private companies. Part C provides the same coverage that is available under Part A and Part B but may also offer additional services; however, Medicare Advantage Plans may have some restrictions, such as the requirement of using physicians in a specific network. Some Advantage plans also include Part D coverage.

**73. A:** If the County Hospital has received an administrative request from a law enforcement official for copies of a patient's records related to a criminal proceeding, according to HIPAA's Privacy Rule, the three criteria that must be met before information is disclosed are:

Relevance: The records provided must directly relate to the criminal proceeding.

Specificity: Only those records related to the proceeding should be released

Identifiable information necessary: Information that has not been de-identified is necessary for the proceeding.

**74. D:** The workload (data) distribution techniques used with a distributed database include fragmentation (horizontal and vertical), allocation, and replication. A distributed database has data stored at different sites and comprises a number of sites connected by a communications network so that each site has its own database system but all sites work together so that data can be accessed at any site. A distributed database is managed by a distributed database management system (DDBMS).

**75. B:** If a hospital is among the 25% of hospitals with the highest rates of hospital-acquired conditions (HACs), the percentage reduction in payment that CMS will impose is 1%. As of 2016, hospitals receive scores ranging from 1 to 10 in two domains: Domain 1 (AHRQ Patient Safety Indicators) and Domain 2 (CDC NHSN Measures). Domain 1 is weighted at 25% and Domain 2 at 75%. Each item in the domains is assigned a score, averaging the scores within the domain to reach a final score. Then, the domain scores are multiplied by the weighted domain percentage and added for the total HAC score.

**76. A:** If a patient's primary diagnosis reads "Renal cell carcinoma of the upper pole of the left kidney, stage 1, grade 2," then the ICD-10-CM code that should be applied is C64.2, indicating the left kidney. "Carcinoma" indicates a type of neoplasm (cancer), and since the involvement is in the "upper pole" or top of the kidney, then the pelvis is not involved. Since the left kidney is specified, the coding with "unspecified urinary organs" does not apply.

**77. C:** The three criteria that electronic signatures must meet when used for medical records are:

Message integrity: The receiver of the medical record should be able to confirm that no alterations were made to the record after the signature was applied.

Nonrepudiation: Once a person signs the record using a distinct signature, the person should not be able to deny having signed the record.

User authentication: The receiver of the medical record should be able to confirm that the person whose signature is applied to the record was the actual person who signed the record.

**78. A:** If a system failure has resulted in corrupted data, the immediate response should be to revert to backup, data stored prior to the system failure. The longer HIM waits to take this action, the more data will have to be reentered, and this can become very time consuming and difficult to manage considering the typical flow of data. Data are vulnerable to corruption during system changes, such as changes in coding systems, so data must be carefully assessed and protected.

**79. C:** If Medicare is to pay for skilled nursing facility care for a patient who was hospitalized as an inpatient in an acute care hospital under Medicare A from March 7 to March 15, the patient must be admitted to the skilled nursing facility within 30 days of discharge. Patients are limited to 100 days of covered care in a skilled nursing facility during a benefit period. Beyond this period of time, the patient is responsible for payment unless the patient has long-term care insurance or is eligible for Medicaid.

**80. C:** The purpose of an Advance Beneficiary Notice is to notify patients that a service may not be covered by Medicare. The services in question should be itemized and the reason provided. The estimated cost of the services should also be included in the notice so that a patient can make an informed decision about whether to proceed and pay for the services. Usually the form has two options: "Yes" to proceed with the services and "No" to not proceed. The form must be dated and signed by the patient.

**81. D:**

| # | Charge code | Item | Price | CPT | Rev code |
|---|---|---|---|---|---|
| 001 | 10006873 | Telemetry Hourly | 300.00 | 99220 | 762 |
| 002 | 10021988 | ICU room charge, Normal | 9112.00 | | 200 |
| 003 | 31068216 | Cardioversion, Defib. | 1820.00 | 92960 | 480 |
| 004 | 31072831 | ECG w/o interp | 765.00 | 93005 | 730 |

According to the charge description master (CDM; also known as chargemaster), if a patient was hospitalized in ICU for 3 days and had hourly telemetry for 24 hours, 4 ECGs, and cardioversion, the amount charged to payers would be $39,416.

$$\text{Telemetry} = \$300 \times 24 = \$7,200$$
$$\text{Room} = \$9112 \times 3 = \$27,336$$
$$\text{ECG} = \$765 \times 4 = \$3,060$$
$$\underline{\text{Cardioversion} = \$1,800}$$
$$\text{Total} = \$39,396$$

**82. B:** According to the six stages of the revenue cycle, after services are provided, the next stage involves documenting services. If a service is not documented, then there is no supporting evidence for the claim. After documentation, the next stage is establishing the charges for the service through manual coding or hardcoding. Then, a bill must be prepared and a claim submitted. The last stage is receiving payment and reconciling the records to show that payment was received.

**83. A:** When utilizing a *charge explosion* system for the chargemaster, five different chargeable processes that are part of one service would be entered into the system under one code, but this code would then expand into the 5 different coded items that compose the service for billing purposes. This essentially bundles the items together to make data entry more efficient. Chargemasters typically list the maximum possible price rather than lower prices that may be negotiated by payers, such as insurance companies. Some chargemasters list different pricing levels.

**84. B:** If a claim for outpatient service is billed to Medicare and outpatient code edits (OCE) result in a claim-level disposition of *suspension*, the healthcare provider must provide requested information. OCE may result in the following claim-level dispositions:

Claim rejected: The healthcare provider must correct the claim prior to resubmission.

Claim denied: The healthcare provider may appeal the decision.

Claim returned to healthcare provider: The healthcare provider must correct problems prior to resubmission.

Claim suspended: The healthcare provider must provide requested information.

**85. D:** If a healthcare provider applies multiple codes, resulting in multiple claims, for a service that should have been covered by one code and one claim, this is an example of unbundling. Unbundling may be done when separate claims result in higher revenue, but this is a fraudulent practice. Upcoding occurs when a healthcare provider assigns a diagnostic or procedure code that results in higher revenue than the appropriate codes. Double billing occurs when the same service is billed for twice.

**86. B:** If the hospital administrator wants to compare the caseloads of different oncologists on the staff and asks the HIM director to prepare a report, the most appropriate place to find that data is the physician index. The physician index lists physicians either in alphabetical order or numerical order (based on the physician's ID number). The listing generally also includes patient's healthcare ID numbers, the diagnoses, admission date, and disposition (discharge, death, transfer). Other demographic information may be included as well.

**87. C:** If information about a well-known patient's physical exam, diagnosis, and treatment is leaked to a local newspaper, the best method to try to determine who leaked the information is likely to conduct an audit trail. This can help to identify users with unauthorized access and to limit the number of possible persons who could have leaked the information. However, it can be difficult to trace leaks if they occur because staff gossip among themselves and because authorized users may allow others to shoulder surf and read from the patient's health record.

**88. D:** If County Hospital wants to decrease the rate of readmissions by providing high-risk patients with case managers, the best method to identify these patients is to use a software application to mine data regarding risk factors from the EHRs. The risk factors must be identified, often by a committee or group of individuals, and may include such risk factors as diagnosis, age, living situation, available resources, and lifestyle choices (smoking, drinking, exercise).

**89. A:** If a hospital has established a facility-based trauma registry, and the 20th patient to be added to the registry was first admitted in May 2015 with a first incidence of trauma, the correct accession number is 15-0020-01. The first number indicates the year (2015), the next set of numbers indicates the sequential order of the visit that year (0020), and the third set of numbers indicates the individual patient's incidences of trauma. In this case, the -01 shows this is the patient's first incidence of trauma.

**90. C:** If a patient was hospitalized for 4 days and then discharged but readmitted 6 days later for a 3-day stay, an interval history and physical exam to cover the period the patient was outside of the hospital and the problems that arose must be done but not a complete history and physical exam as long as the readmission occurs within 30 days. The original history and physical should be included in the new EHR as well.

**91. A:** According to CMS, the three key components when selecting the correct level of E/M services are history, examination, and decision making. There are 4 levels to each of these components, and they are coded and billed differently. The four types of history and examination are problem focused, expanded problem focused, detailed, and comprehensive. The components of a history include chief complaint, history of present illness, review of systems, and past, family, and/or social history. The types of decision making include straightforward, low complexity, moderate complexity, and high complexity.

**92. C:** An example of a finding associated with a qualitative review of an EHR is when the dressing change is not documented for one day because this demonstrates an inconsistency between the physician order and the completion of the order. This finding may indicate an error because the dressing change was missed or it may indicate the failure to document the procedure. Quantitative review identifies missing elements, such as missing signatures or reports.

**93. A:**

| Admission Date | Discharge Date |
| --- | --- |
| May 1 | May 15 |
| July 2 | July 8 |
| August 10 | August 30 |
| September 18 | September 22 |
| October 10 | October 14 |

According to these admission and discharge dates and CMS guidelines, all of these hospitalizations occurred within one benefit period. The patient was initially admitted on May 1, but between that date and the final discharge date on October 14, there was no period in which the patient had no inpatient care for a period of 60 days. Patients can have multiple hospitalizations in one benefit period.

**94. C:** If County Hospital has experienced a flood when a nearby river overflowed during a severe rainstorm, inundating the records room located in the basement and saturating a large volume of records, the best salvage method is to keep the records intact and freeze them at about minus 20°F/-29°C in preparation for a freeze-drying procedure. The records can be sealed in plastic for transfer, but the papers in the files should not be separated, as this is easier to do once the papers are dry.

**95. B:** NDC (National Drug Codes) is the standard data set under HIPAA for pharmacy transactions involving drugs and biologics and is included in Medicare D data. NDCs are product identifiers. Each drug is assigned a number including 3 parts: a labeler/vendor code, a product code, and a trade package code. The NDC Directory is available online as a downloadable file, which is owned by the FDA and distributed by the Department of Health and Human Services.

**96. D:** With ICD-10-CM, injuries are grouped by body part rather than category of injury, as in ICD-9-CM. Thus, all injuries to the thorax (S20-S29) are grouped together. The chapter dealing with injuries, poisoning, and other consequences of external causes are divided by two letters, S and T. The S-coded injuries are grouped by single body regions; however, some injuries are not localized, such as poisonings, and these are T-coded injuries.

**97. C:** According to ICD-10-PCS, if a patient undergoes a thrombectomy to remove a clot from the leg, the root operation for this surgical procedure is *extirpation*. *Excision* is to cut out/off a body part, such as when conducting a biopsy. *Extraction* is pulling or stripping out a body part by force, such as a vein stripping. The term *removal* is used to indicate removing a device from a body part, such as removal of a pacemaker.

**98. A:** As part of denials management, if coding has been missing for some services because physicians frequently forget to document bedside procedures, such as wound care, the best solution may be to provide coders access to account charges. The coders can then look for discrepancy between supplies used and procedures. This also provides the opportunity for the coders to look for missing or misplaced charges.

**99. D:** When an enterprise-wide master patient index (MPI) fails to link two medical files for a patient who has been treated at two participating organizations and the patient ends up with two identifiers in the MPI, this type of error is an overlap. Because of the overlap, a physician accessing the patient's records at one organization would not have access to the records from the other organization. A duplicate occurs if one patient has two identifiers and records within one organization and an overlay if two people have the same identifier.

**100. B:** If a hospital has an average of 450 discharges every month and the number of delinquent records for 1 month is 126, the delinquency rate for the month is 28%. The numerator is the number of delinquent records counted on the last day of the month or predetermined period (not to exceed 30 days). The denominator is the average number of discharges per month.

$$\frac{126}{450} = 0.28 \rightarrow 28\%$$

Delinquency rates should not exceed 50%.

**101. C:** If utilizing an unlisted procedure code for CPT coding for a surgical procedure, a required submission is the operative report. Additional information may also be requested to support the claim. Unlisted codes are utilized when there are no category I or II codes or HCPCS codes that are appropriate. Unlisted codes are found throughout the CPT system and usually conclude with "99." When the unlisted procedure code is used for diagnostic tests, additional submission includes clinical notes with the patient's diagnosis as well as the name of the test and the results.

**102. D:** If an operative report describes procedures as "Complete left mastectomy with insertion of breast prosthesis. Nipple reconstruction began but discontinued when patient's became severely hypotensive," these codes should be applied:

19303-LT (Simple complete mastectomy, left side).

19340-LT (Immediate insertion of breast prosthesis following mastopexy, mastectomy, on in reconstruction, left side).

19350-53-LT (Nipple/areola reconstruction, procedure discontinued, left side).

**103. C:** If a patient had a skin tag removed on March 1 and returned to the same physician on March 3 for a laceration repair unrelated to the first surgery, the patient would be covered under the Medicare's global surgical package for the minor surgical procedures for a total of 13 days. Two days would be covered for the first procedure, the day of surgery and the following day, but that time period stops when the second one starts. Eleven days are covered for the second procedure, the day of the surgery and the next 10 days.

**104. A:** Although the child was brought to the emergency department, the child's injuries are not likely life-threatening or severe because the child was able to walk on the injured leg. The emergency department physician should conduct only a medical screening examination and then wait for consent from the parents before conducting further tests or providing treatment. A friend of the family has no legal right to grant consent, and a court order is not warranted for a minor injury.

**105. D:** While ensuring financial goals is always a concern, it is not a critical role for the HIM department to play in data standardization. The HIM department should identify key elements requiring standardization by ensuring that all key elements are included in the data dictionary and that definitions are uniform. The HIM department should be actively involved in clinical documentation improvement functions in order to improve the quality of claims and reimbursement and should understand national data standards and ensure they are applied within the organization and should, if possible, participate in the development of data standards.

**106. B:** Considering the domains of quality management, *application* refers to the purpose of the collection of data, how the data will be utilized. *Collection* refers to the manner in which data are collected, all of the steps involved in the process. *Warehousing* refers to the storage and archiving of data and should include security measures to prevent breaches of confidentiality. *Analysis* refers to the manner in which data are translated into information that can be utilized by an application.

**107. C:** Submitting a surgical procedure code can trigger the requirement to report cross-cutting measures to CMS for PQRS. Submitting a claim for a face-to-face encounter is the triggering mechanism, and face-to-face encounters can include outpatient visits and office visits but does not count telehealth visits. Cross-cutting measures are quality measures that apply across different types of healthcare settings and different types of eligible providers and group practices, such as carrying out mediation reconciliation and asking patients about advance care plans.

**108. B:** The primary responsibility when reviewing a physician's credentials is to determine if the person is properly credentialed and has received the appropriate education and meets any other requirements, such as maintaining liability insurance, but quality of care should also be a concern, so any information found in the credentialing process that brings quality of care into question should be referred to the appropriate authority, such as the peer review committee or the chief medical official.

**109. B:** An external audit of coding practices should be conducted at least yearly. Consultants who specialize in conducting audits are brought in to analyze the operations, detect any gaps in performance, and identify problems. Prior to the audit, the HIM director should establish clear goals, secure support from administration, prepare coding professionals, and identify the types of cases to be reviewed. Findings should be reviewed and recommendations implemented.

**110. D:** The correct ICD-10-CM codes are H65.04 (Nonsuppurative acute serous otitis media, recurrent, right ear) and Z77.22 (Exposure to environmental tobacco smoke). Even though the physician did not include "recurrent" in the diagnosis, an episode of bilateral otitis media was recorded as occurring 6 months previously. Because there is no drainage from the ear, the otitis media is "nonsuppurative" rather than "suppurative." H65.04 would be listed first as it is the primary diagnosis.

**111. C:** Although there are some exceptions for mental health patients (such as not providing psychotherapy notes), generally patients have the right to access all of their healthcare records; however, if the requests are extensive, the hospital has the right to charge reasonable copying fees. According to HIPAA requirements, the copies of the record must be provided within 30 days at most. Patients have the right to ask that errors in their records be corrected.

**112. D:** If an RHIT receives a subpoena duces tecum, the technician is being directed to bring records (copies or original) to a legal proceeding, usually a deposition. The subpoena should specify exactly which documents or images are wanted. Because state laws vary, the RHIT should verify responsibilities in regard to responding. A subpoena ad testificandum is directing the RHIT to appear to testify that records are authentic (not altered or incomplete).

**113. A:** In preparation for an HHS Office of Civil Rights (OCR) HIPAA audit, an organization should begin by completing a risk assessment. This includes reviewing all requirements for compliance. The security of PHI must be assessed as well as the type and effectiveness of security controls. Security risks should be identified and prioritized according to the likelihood that a breach could occur and the severity of that breach. The organization should also review all policies regarding privacy and breach notification.

**114. A:**

| ICD-9-CM | Description | ICD-10-CM | Description | Approximate |
|---|---|---|---|---|
| 281.2 | Folate deficiency anemia | D52.0 | Dietary folate deficiency anemia | 1 |
| 281.2 | Folate deficiency anemia | D52.1 | Drug-induced folate deficiency anemia | 1 |
| 281.2 | Folate deficiency anemia | D52.8 | Other folate deficiency anemias | 1 |
| 281.2 | Folate deficiency anemia | D52.9 | Folate deficiency anemia, unspecified. | 1 |

Based on the General Equivalence Mapping above, ICD-9-CM code 281.2 maps approximately to four different ICD-10-CM codes: D52.0, D52.1, D52.8, and D52.9.

**115. A:** If the HIM director is responsible for conducting an internal coding audit, the first step should be to determine the scope of the audit, including the type of services to audit and whether to do the audit retrospectively or prospectively in relation to filing claims. A baseline audit may be conducted to help to determine the scope. Then, the individuals who will conduct the audit should be identified and materials (such as coding manuals) gathered and decisions made about supplementary items (such as charge tickets and claim forms) needed.

**116. D:** If the predicted number of surgical site infections for a hospital is 15, but 26 patients developed surgical site infections, the standardized infection ratio (SIR) is 1.73 (26/15). This indicates that the hospital experienced approximate 73% more infections than was predicted for the size and type of hospital based on national data. A SIR value of less than 1 indicates that the infection rate is less than predicted while a SIR value of more than 1 indicates the infection rate is higher.

**117. B:** Knowledge discovery in databases (KDD) is a method utilized to search databases in order to identify patterns and relationships. KDD is commonly used as a tool of research and includes data mining methods (including decision tree, nonlinear regression, classification, and relational) to extract knowledge. With KDD, data are selected, preprocessed, mined, and interpreted. The primary goal of KDD is to draw conclusions about data.

**118. C:** Only a physician (or other practitioner, such as a nurse practitioner) who provides direct supervision can file a CMS for "incident to" services provided by auxiliary personnel. The supervising healthcare provider may, in fact, be different from the patient's physician or the physician who ordered the service. Auxiliary personnel may be employees, independent contractors, or leased employees, and they must meet any state requirement (such as licensure) required for the service provided.

**119. C:** Following FDA approval of an item and during the time when a new code is being considered for this item through the HCPCS review process, the type of HCPCS level II code that should be utilized is a miscellaneous code. Miscellaneous codes are used when there is no national code that is appropriate for the item or service. Documentation regarding the claim should be submitted to the payer. Temporary codes are those assigned by insurers before the next code update or when a consensus about coding the item or service has not been reached.

**120. D:** If a 70-year-old patient came to the emergency department for a right wrist injury, an x-ray showed a non-displaced Colles fracture, and a short arm prefabricated splint was applied, the following codes would be utilized:

Diagnosis: ICD-10-CM.

X-ray: CPT.

Splint (includes application): HCPCS level II L code.

No manipulation was required because the fracture was non-displaced. A CPT code for application of a splint is only utilized if the splint is specifically made and fitted to the patient, but, in this case, a prefabricated splint was used, and application is included in the L code for the splint.

**121. D:** If a neoplasm is described with the term "adenoma," "lipoma," "fibroma" or "nevi," then the RHIT should use the "benign" column in the ICD-10-CM Table of Neoplasm to identify the correct code because these terms refer to non-malignant lesions. However, if the description includes the word "malignant" or "cancerous," such as "malignant adenoma," then the diagnosis should be coded as a malignancy.

**122. A:** If a patient has a primary diagnosis of prostatic cancer (C61) but is receiving radiation treatment (Z51.0) for metastasis to the bones (C79.51), the therapy would be listed as the principle diagnostic code followed by the metastasis (C79.51), which is the focus of this treatment. The primary diagnosis of prostatic cancer (C61) would be next in the sequence followed by the chronic condition, diabetes mellitus with polyneuropathy (E11.42). Coding sequence:

Z51.0, C79.51, C61, and E11.42.

**123. A:** The NDC that is in the correct format for filing a CMS claim for a drug administered to a patient in an outpatient clinic is 21695-0245-20. NDC codes contain a labeler code, product code, and package code with these three sub-codes separated by a hyphen. The configuration may be 4-4-2 (4 labeler code numbers, 4 product code numbers, and 2 package code numbers), 5-5-2, 5-4-1, or 5-4-2. To comply with HIPAA standards, CMS requires the 5-4-2 (11 digit) code configuration and utilizes leading zeroes if the code has fewer than 11 digits.

**124. A:** If a patient's diagnosis is "MRSA [methicillin-resistant *Staphylococcus aureus*] septicemia," supporting documentation in the form of blood culture and sensitivities should be in the EHR. The blood culture should be positive for the organism and the sensitivity negative for response to methicillin. The complete blood cell count is also supporting but less specific because it can demonstrate the presence of infection (elevated white blood cell count) but provides no information about the organism or resistance to antibiotics.

**125. D:** Providing care for maintenance or caregiver convenience is not a criteria for medical necessity and is not generally covered by Medicare or secondary insurance companies. Criteria include care that is appropriate to the patient's diagnosis, needs, and condition, care provided to restore health or prevent deterioration of health, care provided within clinically accepted medical practice standards, and care provided to prevent a likely health problem or diagnose a problem.

**126. B:** If the same information about a patient is entered into more than one table in a database, this is an example of data redundancy. Data redundancy in a database can pose problems if it is done accidentally because if one table is updated and another is not, this results in data inconsistency where data that should be the same are different. Data redundancy may also be done purposefully as part of backup to ensure that data can be recovered.

**127. A:** A Voluntary Data Sharing Agreement (VDSA) with CMS provides electronic exchange of health benefit information to simplify coordination of healthcare benefit payments between employers and Medicare. Each quarter, the employer forwards group health entitlement information to CMS's Benefits Coordination and Recovery Center, and Medicare, in turn, provides the employer information that identifies group health plan members who are eligible for Medicare benefits.

**128. B:** If, under HIPAA's Security Rule, a healthcare organization determines that an "addressable" implementation specification is not applicable or appropriate for the organization, the healthcare organization must document the decision and the rationale behind it. Additionally, the organization must explain how the standard is met. While implementation specifications are labeled as "required" or "addressable," "addressable" does not mean that the specification is optional. In all cases, the standard must be met in some way.

**129. C:** The TRICARE program that is an HMO style plan is TRICARE Prime. TRICARE Prime can cover not only active duty service members but also retirees from active duty or military reserves who are 60 years and older and their eligible family members. Enrollees select a primary care physician who can provide a referral to specialists. Because of the restrictions in access to physicians, the copayment is small, and those on active duty and their families are not required to pay a fee for enrollment.

**130. D:** If a database notes that a field is empty and displays an error message to remind the user to complete the field, this is an example of a completeness check. The purpose of this type of alert is to ensure that all data are complete. Data must be complete in order to meet the needs of those accessing the data at a future time. Incomplete data may result in important data being omitted from a query or from reports.

**131. D:** If a patient is hospitalized under Medicare twice in 1 year for periods of 92 days and 106 days and 60 days separated the discharge from the first hospitalization to the admission for the second, the patient has used lifetime reserve days for both hospitalizations. Since the lifetime reserve is 90 days, the patient owes for 2 days ($92 - 90 = 2$) for the first hospitalization and 16 days ($106 - 90 = 16$) for the second, for a total of 18 days:

$$18 \times 644 = \$11,592$$

**132. C:** If a MS-DRG has a relative weight of 4.000 compared with a MS-DRG with a relative weight of 2.000, the 4.000 relative weight generally requires twice the resources of the 2.000. The relative weight is assigned to reflect the average resources required in relation to the national average. Hospitals receive reimbursement based on the MS-DRG assigned with each MS-DRG including a description, a relative weight, a mean LOS, and an arithmetic LOS.

**133. B:** If Hospital A and Hospital B both serve the same community, have 450 beds, discharge approximately the same number of patients, and have similar services but Hospital A has a CMI of 1.57 and Hospital B has a CMI of 0.98, the most likely reason for the difference is that Hospital B is not coding or capturing levels of severity (MCC, CC, no-CC) adequately. The higher the CMI, the lower the costs, and vice versa.

**134. C:** Under APC (Ambulatory Payment Classification) guidelines, to qualify for outlier payments, the cost must exceed 2.5 times the APC payment. Any amount below that is considered a normal fluctuation and no additional payment is made. If, for example, costs exceed APC payment by $400, then the outlier payment would be $300 (75% of excess cost). Outlier is an exception to the usual fixed payment rates. Other exceptions are made for pass-through items and new technology.

**135. D:** When calculating the case mix index, the required data include the relative weight of each MS-DRG and the number of discharges in the MS-DRG. The total weight for each MS-DRG is calculated by multiplying the relative weight by the number of discharges. The total weights of all of the MS-DRGs are added together and that number is divided by the total number of discharges in order to obtain the case mix index.

**136. B:**

| Patient A/R Report | | | Days outstanding | | | | | |
|---|---|---|---|---|---|---|---|---|
| ID | Name | Current | 31-60 | 91-120 | 121-150 | 151-180 | 180+ | Total |
| 001 | Doe, J | | | | | | 28.56 | 28.56 |
| 708 | Jones, M | | 42.88 | | | 663.00 | | 705.88 |
| 889 | Lee, J | 178.00 | 217.00 | | 128.78 | | | 523.78 |
| 997 | Jong, M | | | 2850.00 | | 526.42 | | 3376.42 |
| 662 | Brown, A | | | 1066.10 | | | 2896.00 | 3962.10 |
| Totals: | | 178.00 | 259.88 | 3916.10 | 128.78 | 1189.42 | 2924.56 | 8596.74 |

According to the A/R report, the greatest percentage of aged bills occurs in the 91 to 120 days period. Out of the total of unpaid bills ($8596.74), $3916.10 represents 45.5% of the total (3916.10/8596.74). Therefore, the focus on collection should be on these large bills. Small bills, such as the $28.56 that is 180+ days outstanding, should often be written off the books to save time and the expense of repeated billing.

**137. D:** According to the SNF Consolidated Billing (CB) requirement, all PT, OT and SLP services received by the patient must be included on the Part A bill for Medicare-covered services even if the services are provided by an outside entity. SNF CB is the "bundling" requirement for SNFs. While services not directly provided were at one time billed separately by the outside entity providing the service, this resulted in many duplicate claims.

**138. B:** After a claim is entered into a payer's system, the action that occurs next is that the claim information is reviewed against the payer's data file in order to determine if coverage is active and was active at the time the service was provided. The claim is reviewed to ensure preauthorization requirements were met and the LOS was appropriate. Once this is completed, computerized edits are conducted to determine if any procedure was inappropriate for age or gender, and to ensure procedures were medically necessary and that bundled services were not unbundled. Then a payment determination is made and payment sent.

**139. A:** The three types of edits that are carried out by the Medicare Code Editor (MCE) are:

Inpatient coding: Ensures diagnosis/procedures codes are correct and that the 4th or 5th digit of the diagnosis code is correct. Checks for age and gender conflicts and ensures principal diagnosis matches claim for services.

Coverage: Ensures procedure is covered and completes Medicare secondary payer (MSP) alert.

Inpatient Clinical: Checks for bilateral procedures, validity of age and gender, and valid discharge status.

**140. B:** In the Medicare appeals process, the order of appeals is as follows:

Redetermination: Claims reviewed by a different Medicare Administrative Contractor (MAC).

Reconsideration: Case reconsidered by a Qualified Independent Contractor (QIC).

Hearing: Case reviewed at a hearing before an Administrative Law Judge (ALJ)

Review: Medicare Appeals Council reviews the case.

Judicial review: Case goes to the US District Court.

**141. D:** According to the federal False Claims Act, if a provider bills Medicare $250 for services that were not provided to the patient and later submits another claim for $125 for services not provided, the fine would be $21,125. The fine is 3 times the billed amounts plus $10,000 for *each* claim:

$$\$250 + \$125 = \$375 \times 3 = \$1125$$

$$\$1125 + \$20,000 = \$21,125$$

The False Claims Act includes a provision providing a reward for people who report fraudulent claims (whistleblowers).

**142. C:** If a healthcare organization shows a profit of $120,000 on $2 million dollars in revenue, the organization's profit margin is 6% ($120,000/$2,000,000 = 0.06). The goal of managing a budget is to have a positive profit margin, although healthcare organizations, such as hospitals, often run very low or negative profit margins with the average profit margins for hospitals under 8%. When profit margins are low, the solution often focuses on cost-cutting measures.

**143. C:** According to the chart regarding complaints about the EHR system, approximately 55 complaints were made about the system being slow and 38 complaints were about log-in problems. Because both of these issues have to do with system performance, the action that is most indicated is to conduct system testing to identify problems and improve performance.

**144. A:** In the conversion from paper records to the EHR, back-scanning is often done. Back-scanning is scanning in paper records that are already in existence so that they can be accessed electronically. For example, a HIM department may decide to back-scan only the previous year's records or may decide to begin scanning records only at a future point in the conversion project. Back-scanning saves physical storage space but may increase costs of digital storage.

**145. B:** The best method of establishing productivity goals for coding professionals is to measure actual production over a specified period of time, usually at least 4 to 6 weeks. Once statistics have been gathered and compiled, the average for the group as a whole should be calculated. Because this rate is affected by outliers, such as a staff person with very low productivity, an additional average of that average productivity rate of the group and the rate of most productive worker should provide a reasonable, but not too easy, goal.

**146. D:** If, as part of the clinical documentation management program (CDMP) to improve documentation of medical necessity and decrease coding errors at a large teaching hospital, coders have been assigned to teams to code for specialty units, such as oncology and cardiac care, the next step should be to provide specialty unit-specific training. This training should include a review of medical terminology, common diagnoses, symptoms, and treatments. Coders should meet with unit healthcare providers in order to establish working relationships.

**147. A:** If using CPT code 20680 (removal of implant, deep) for a hardware removal procedure after a physician removed a plate and 3 screws from an orthopedic injury because of a metal sensitivity reaction, the code should be entered on the claim form only one time. Even though 4 pieces of hardware were removed, the removal was done during one procedure. CPT code 20680 should be used only if the removal involves an incision through multiple layers of tissue. Superficial removals should be coded 20670.

**148. D:** A healthcare facility should retain the register of surgical procedures permanently. While most records are maintained for 10 years, and diagnostic images and mammography for 5 years, some records should be maintained permanently, including registers of births and deaths, and the master patient index. However, there are no clear national regulations regarding retention, and state requirements may vary.

**149. C:** While registered nurses (RNs) can carry out orders, they cannot legally diagnose or write medical orders; however, a registered nurse with specialized education, such as a nurse practitioner (NP), can do so. Physician assistants (PAs) may also be allowed to diagnose and write orders. In some states, NPs and PAs require some type of physician supervision, and there may be limitations to the types of medical orders that they can write.

**150. B:** If the master patient index (MPI) includes a *Soundex* field, the name "Parker" would be coded P626. The code starts with the first letter of the person's name followed by codes that correspond to the consonants in the name. If the digital code is less than 3 digits long, then an ending 0 is added. For longer names, the coding stops with 3 digits. *Soundex* files may be used to look up a file if the spelling of the person's name is unknown.

**151. C:** If a healthcare provider's fee is $180, but the provider has agreed to a write-down adjustment of $40 from the insurance company, this results in a negotiated fee of $140 per visit ($180 − $40). However, the insurance company pays only 75% of the negotiated price, $140 × 0.75 = $105.00. The patient's copayment is $140 × 0.25 = $35.00. A provider may have a fee scale with a number of different fees based on different contractual agreements.

**152. A:** A "bill-hold period" is typically used by HIM to ensure that all charges are posted on the claim before it is submitted. This period may vary but is typically relatively short, about 3 to 5 days after discharge. During this time, the coding of the record should be completed. However, if the record is incomplete, coding may take longer, and rushing to finish may result in missed codes and lower rates of reimbursement.

**153. A:** The purpose of grouper software is to classify patients into the correct MS-DRG based on ICD-10-CM code, severity of illness, and risk of mortality. Healthcare organizations often purchase software that updates when changes are made and integrates with other information systems. Grouper software is able to calculate expected reimbursement so that the healthcare organization can budget accordingly. While it is possible to manually assign MS-DRGs, doing so is very complex because there are many factors to consider.

**154. B:** When a claim is submitted to CMS, the factors that affect the MS-DRG reimbursement are the relative weight assigned an MS-DRG and the hospital IPPS rate. The relative weight reflects the average relative cost of a group's cases compared with the cost of the average Medicare case. For example, some MS-DRGs, such as transplants, are weighted very highly because their cost of care is much higher than the average Medicare patient's care.

**155. B:** In a transaction-processing system (TPS), a detailed report about admissions would be classified as a *product*. Data from different types of products may be used to make staffing or other decisions. TPS manages various types of transactions that are common in healthcare organizations. Transactions can include such things as admissions and supply purchases. TPS includes inputs and outputs. Users are generally those involved in making operational decisions, such as managers or supervisors at lower levels.

**156. C:** For the Medicare fee schedule that lists allowable charges for physicians under Medicare B, the factors that are utilized when calculating relative value units (RVUs) and geographic practice cost indices (GPCIs) include:

Physician work: Time and intensity of services provided to patients.

Practice expenses: Includes both direct costs (staff labor, medical equipment, medical supplies) and indirect costs.

Malpractice costs: Cost of malpractice insurance premiums according to specialty.

**157. D:** In the OPPS, an "N" status indicator means that the item or service is packaged into the APC (ambulatory payment classification) group of another service/item, so no separate payment will be received. Services/Items that are packaged may include minor medications, medical supplies, and devices. CMS assigns a status indicator to each HCPCS/CPT code, indicating how the service/item will be reimbursed. Status indicators A, B, C, and D all indicate services or items that will not receive reimbursement, for various reasons.

**158. B:** If further information is needed to complete coding of a patient's record and the physician must be queried, the most efficient method is usually to send a query form because it can contain detailed information and cover specific questions. For example, if a number of abnormal findings are documented on the history and physical with no corresponding diagnosis, these findings can be documented on the query. Query forms may be transmitted electronically or on paper.

**159. A:** With medical and surgical procedures in ICD-10-PCS, the seven characters utilized for coding include the following meanings:

| 1 | 2 | 3 | 4 | 5 | 6 | 7 |
|---|---|---|---|---|---|---|
| Section | Body system | Root operation | Body part | Approach | Device | Qualifier |

Section: General type of procedure

Body system: Indicated by numbers ore letters.

Root operations: 31 different procedures.

Body part: Indicated by number or letter according to body system.

Approach: Varies according to body part but may include open, percutaneous, via natural or artificial opening, and via natural or artificial opening endoscopic.

Device: Z is used to designate NO device

Qualifier: Z indicates NO qualifier.

**160. C:** If a PCP in an HMO receives payment based on *capitation* (head count), this means that the physician receives a flat fee based on the number of patients in the HMO who have selected the physician as his/her physician, whether or not the physician actually provides care to the patient. This method is most effective with large groups of HMO patients because some patients will need extensive care and some none.

**161. D:** If two hospitals each have the same number of licensed beds but the first hospital (X) has an ALOS of 3 and discharges 30,000 patients per year and the second hospital (Y) has an ALOS of 6 and discharges 15,000 per year, the first hospital (X) has the greater capacity because the lower ALOS allows the hospital to serve more patients with the same number of beds. Capacity may be assessed either according to the number of licensed beds or through comparing the ALOS and the discharges.

**162. D:** A part of utilization management, intensity-of-service and severity of illness (ISSI) screening criteria are used to determine whether a patient requires inpatient or outpatient care. This type of screening is often used to decide if a patient's surgical procedure should be done as an outpatient or an inpatient. Severity-of-illness screening determines whether a patient needs inpatient care based on physical impairment. Continued-stay/concurrent utilization determines whether a patient needs continued inpatient care or care at the same level. Prospective utilization determines whether inpatient care is a medical necessity.

**163. B:** If physicians and nursing staff persistently use workarounds to the EHR, such as copying and pasting information and writing information and orders on paper for later entries, resulting in medical errors, the most common reason for workarounds is that the EHR design is incompatible with work processes. Problems can include slow access time, data entry not reflecting needs, too many steps involved in a process, and computer stations for entry not available at the point of care.

**164. B:** When conducting testing on health information technology projects in the health information management department, testing should be done in the following order:

(1) Unit: Testing of individual components and programs.

(2) Integration: Testing to determine how system subsets work together.

(3) System: Testing of the entire system.

(4) Usability: Testing by end users to determine if the system fits workflow and other end-user needs.

**165. A:** The OASIS-C1 (Outcomes and Assessment Information Set) is a standardized data set designed to gather data about Medicare patients who are under the care of a home health agency. OASIS-C1 is the version developed for use with ICD-10-CM. OASIS data about a patient's condition and therapy needs are used to determine the case-mix adjustment to the base payment rate. HHA providers complete an HH patient tracking sheet that includes CMS certification number, NPI, and patient demographic information, as well as the date of start of care and resumption of care and current payment source for HH care.

# Practice Test #2

**1. The Medicare Outpatient Code Editor (OCE) conducts the following types of edits: coding, coverage, clinical, and**

    a. claims.
    b. coverage.
    c. cancellation.
    d. cause.

**2. When calculating the fetal death rate for the hospital, which of the following should be included in the calculations?**

    a. All fetal deaths, regardless of weeks of gestation or weight
    b. All fetal deaths occurring at or after 20 weeks' gestation or weight of at least 501 g
    c. All fetal deaths occurring at or after 10 weeks' gestation
    d. Only fetal deaths occurring at or after 28 weeks' gestation or weight of greater than 1000 g

**3. If an insurer, such as Blue Cross/Blue Shield, denies a claim, within how many days of denial must an internal appeal be submitted?**

    a. 30
    b. 60
    c. 90
    d. 180

**4. Which of the following is an example of malware that copies itself and spreads throughout a system?**

    a. Computer virus
    b. Trojan horse
    c. Computer worm
    d. Rootkit

**5. A patient receives care from a physician who is a non-participating Medicare provider who does not accept assignment, and the actual charge for the visit is $300. However, the usual, customary, and reasonable (UCR) charge is $240.00, and the patient has no supplementary insurance. How much out-of-pocket cost will the patient incur?**

    a. $108.00
    b. $117.60
    c. $48.40
    d. $60.00

**6. A patient's primary insurance company requires both a deductible and copayments for outpatient services:**

**Patient's financial responsibilities.**

| Deductible | $150 annually |
|---|---|
| Office visits | $20 copayment |
| Laboratory tests | $5 copayment per lab test |
| CT, MRI, PET scan | $25 copayment per test |
| X-ray | $10 copayment per order |
| ED visit | $100 copayment |

**Over the course of a year, the patient received a number of outpatient services. What total amount is the patient's financial responsibility?**

**Patient's medical expenses**

| Service | Unit cost | Unit # | Total cost |
|---|---|---|---|
| Office visits (OV) | $110.00 | 8 | $880.00 |
| Laboratory tests | Varies | 10 | 285.00 |
| MRI | 1500.00 | 1 | 1500.00 |
| ED visit | 600.00 | 1 | 600.00 |
| X-ray | 120.00 | 1 | 120.00 |
| TOTAL | | | $3385.00 |

- a. $345.00
- b. $395.00
- c. $445.00
- d. $495.00

**7. If a healthcare organization wants a classification system to quantify levels of functional ability and disability, which of the following is the best option?**

- a. LOINC
- b. ICPC
- c. ICF
- d. ICD-O

**8. A patient is being treated specifically with antineoplastic immunotherapy (Z51.12) for multiple myeloma (C90.00), which has not yet achieved remission. The patient also has a history of supraventricular tachycardia (I46.1), controlled by medication. How would these diagnoses be sequenced, first to last?**

- a. Z51.12, C90.00, and I46.1
- b. I46.1, C90.00, and Z51.12
- c. I46.1, Z51.12, C90.00
- d. C90.00, Z51.12, and I46.1

9. When calculating the readmission adjustment factor (RAF) for MS-DRG base rate, if the base operating DRG is $5040 and the readmission adjustment factor is 0.9990 less 1.0, the adjustment to the base rate is

    a. +$5.04
    b. (−$5.04)
    c. +$4.03
    d. (−$4.03)

10. When billing for dental claims, which coding system is utilized?

    a. CPT
    b. ICD-10-PCS
    c. NDC
    d. CDT

11. In HCPCS level II codes, which type of code would be used for drugs that are not administered orally, such as chemotherapy drugs and inhalational drugs?

    a. A codes
    b. D codes
    c. E codes
    d. J codes

12. Forms control is a process in which

    a. information is entered into the computer.
    b. records holding patient information are protected.
    c. specific forma are created for specific purposes.
    d. documents are imaged.

13. The purpose of a clinical pertinence review is to

    a. ensure documentation is appropriate.
    b. institute disciplinary procedures.
    c. determine if forms require modification to meet standards.
    d. compare physicians' competency levels.

14. One procedure always involves 5 separate charges, but errors in coding for the charges frequently result in omission of one or two charges. The best solution may be to

    a. post directions for staff members.
    b. utilize a charge explosion code.
    c. institute disciplinary measures.
    d. have entry of one code trigger a reminder alert.

15. A patient was hospitalized in the psychiatric unit for 60 days following a suicide attempt. The insurance company has requested a copy of the psychiatrist's psychotherapy notes. The correct response is to

    a. send a copy of the notes.
    b. ask the psychiatrist for permission to send the notes.
    c. refer the request to the ethics committee.
    d. decline to send a copy of the notes.

**16. The *guarantor* of an account is the**

    a. insurance company that will provide payment for claims.

    b. the person for whom the account is established.

    c. the person who is responsible for paying bills not paid for by insurance.

    d. the person show is responsible for signing consent forms.

**17. When should the RHIT expect an organization to begin to prepare for accreditation review by The Joint Commission?**

    a. Every day

    b. A year before the review

    c. A month before the review

    d. When new standards are issued

**18. The primary difference between licensed beds in a facility and the bed count is that the bed count is the**

    a. actual number of beds in a facility.

    b. number of beds that are ready for patients and staffed.

    c. number of beds that have been approved for the facility by the state.

    d. number of beds that actually are assigned to patients.

**19. Over a 7-day period, 25 people were discharged from the oncology unit of hospital. The lengths of stay were as follows:**

        15 patients: 4 days

        1 patient: 20 days

        4 patients: 2 days

        5 patients: 1 day

        1 patient: 7 days

**What is the average length of stay (ALOS) in the oncology unit?**

    a. 3 days

    b. 4 days

    c. 5 days

    d. 6 days

**20. If a patient is treated in the emergency department for 2 hours and then kept for observation in a special unit adjacent to the emergency department for 36 hours following a concussion and episodes of confusion, how is the patient classified?**

    a. Outpatient for 2 hours and inpatient for 36 hours

    b. Outpatient for 24 hours and inpatient for 12 hours

    c. Inpatient for the entire stay

    d. Outpatient for the entire stay

21. Community Hospital began the year with an average length of stay of 4.9 in January and has instituted efficiency measures to try to decrease the ALOS to at least 4. Comparing figures, how effective has the hospital been in reducing the ALOS?

**Average Length of Stay by Department over a 6-Month Period**

| Dept. | Jan | Feb | March | April | May | June |
|--------|------|------|-------|-------|------|------|
| Med. | 5 | 5.2 | 4.8 | 4.7 | 4.9 | 5 |
| Surg. | 5.6 | 5.8 | 5.3 | 5.5 | 5.4 | 5.3 |
| Onc. | 5.0 | 4.8 | 5.1 | 4.9 | 5.2 | 4.8 |
| Ped. | 3.6 | 3.8 | 3.4 | 3.5 | 3.7 | 3.6 |
| OB-Gyn | 3.2 | 3.4 | 3.0 | 3.6 | 3.1 | 3.3 |
| Psych. | 7.2 | 7.5 | 7.3 | 7.2 | 7.7 | 7.4 |

    a. There has been almost no change.
    b. The ALOS has increased.
    c. The ALOS has decreased.
    d. Some departments have shown marked improvement.

22. Which of the following is NOT classified as a clinical allied health professional?

    a. OT
    b. RT
    c. RN
    d. PT

23. The size of an outpatient facility is determined by its

    a. licensed beds.
    b. bed count.
    c. visits/encounters per day.
    d. square feet of facility.

24. In order to comply with accreditation standards of TJC, following admission to an acute care facility, a complete history and physical examination must be completed for an inpatient within how many hours?

    a. 2 hours
    b. 6 hours
    c. 12 hours
    d. 24 hours

25. PHI refers to

    a. personal health information.
    b. protected health information.
    c. private health information.
    d. primary health information.

26. The American College of Surgeons first developed a health initiative that required hospitals to keep records of care and treatment in what year?

    a. 1948
    b. 1938
    c. 1928
    d. 1918

**27. Under HIPAA's Privacy Rule, *consent* is for**
  a. treatment.
  b. storage of PHI.
  c. use of PHI.
  d. marketing of PHI.

**28. Which of the following is a *physical* safeguard of the security standards in HIPAA?**
  a. Restricted access to EPHI
  b. Authentication controls
  c. Encryption/Decryption
  d. Delegation of security response

**29. In the relational database below, what are the foreign key or keys in table 2?**

Table 1
**Customers**

| ID # | Last name | First name | Street | City, State, Zip |
|---|---|---|---|---|
| 001 | Johnson | Mark | 240 West St. | SF, CA, 94101 |
| 002 | Smith | Maria | 180 Sanctum Ct. | PA, CA, 94062 |
| 003 | Masters | Sue | 355 James Way | SJ, CA, 95038 |

Table 2
**Medical Supply Orders**

| Order # | Order date | Customer ID # | Product # | # Units |
|---|---|---|---|---|
| 01 | 01-16-16 | 002 | 2680 | 2 |
| 02 | 01-17-16 | 001 | 2682 | 1 |
| 03 | 01-17-16 | 003 | 2681 | 4 |

Table 3
**Medical Supplies**

| Product # | Name | Price per unit |
|---|---|---|
| 2680 | Silicone foam dressings | $30.00 |
| 2681 | Surgical gauze pads | $7.00 |
| 2682 | Petrolatum dressings | $66.00 |

  a. Order # and Customer ID #
  b. Customer ID # and Product #
  c. Customer ID #
  d. Order #

**30. In ACSII, bytes with a value of 32 to 126 are used to represent**

    a. numbers, letters, and punctuation.
    b. extended characters.
    c. images.
    d. audio files.

**31. In a database, which of the following comprises groups of fields?**

    a. Files
    b. Tables
    c. Records
    d. Characters

**32. Images, such as MRI images, CT images, and x-rays are captured and stored in a database according to which of the following standards?**

    a. ASCII
    b. PDF
    c. DICOM
    d. TIFF

**33. *Payment floor* refers to**

    a. a negotiated payment that is less that the standard charge for healthcare services.
    b. the time period when Medicare/insurance companies delay sending reimbursement after adjudication.
    c. a payment for outlier charges that are lower than usual payments.
    d. a list of charge items that are no longer utilized but still in the chargemaster.

**34. A healthcare organization plans to use software applications from different vendors as part of its new electronic health record, but each application requires the user to log in. What should be implemented to allow the user to log in to all the different applications at the same time?**

    a. IMAP
    b. POP3
    c. DICOM
    d. CCOM

35. A large healthcare organization has invested in a new software application to improve billing procedures with an initial outlay of $250,000 and $120,000 the second year followed by ongoing maintenance and upgrade costs. The organization expects an immediate payback on investment. The graph above shows the cumulative costs and benefits. At what point did payback on investment occur?

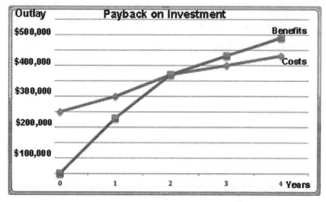

a. Year 1
b. Year 2
c. Year 3
d. Year 4

36. Which of the following is NOT an example of a primary health record?

a. Acute care electronic health record
b. Physician office patient chart
c. Health insurance claims
d. Home health agency patient record

37. With the ICD-10-PCS procedure code, which letters are NOT used?

a. I and O
b. Q and X
c. Y and Z
d. O and Q

38. Which of the following data sets are required by CMS for long-term care facilities?

a. OASIS-CI
b. UCDS
c. DEEDS
d. RAI

39. According to AHIMA's recommended minimum retention periods, how long should adult health records be retained?

a. 5 years
b. 10 years
c. 15 years
d. 20 years

**40. Which of the following is a secondary purpose of the electronic health record?**

    a. Documentation of services received
    b. Fostering continuity of care
    c. Serving as evidence in litigation
    d. Verification of billing

**41. Upon review of a patient's electronic health record, it is noted that a rash on the patient's torso is described by different healthcare providers as "macular," "papular," "measles-like," "red," "raised," and "allergic." Which of the following quality characteristics of data quality management does this violate?**

    a. Data consistency
    b. Data accuracy
    c. Data precision
    d. Data definition

**42. Which system of numbering for charts is used when a patient is assigned a number on a first admission to a hospital and is assigned the same number with each subsequent admission?**

    a. Unit
    b. Serial
    c. Family
    d. Serial unit

**43. Which of the following is NOT found in a diagnostic report?**

    a. Laboratory tests, such as BUN
    b. Heart tracing (electrocardiogram)
    c. Microscopic analysis of tissue sample
    d. Description of anesthesia

**44. The Security Management Process for HIPAA's Security Management Standard begins with which implementation?**

    a. Sanction policy
    b. Risk management
    c. Information system activity review
    d. Risk analysis

**45. If using SQL to query a relational database with the headings as in the table below, what is the correct query for a list of the names of RNs only, including their employee IDs?**

**Employees**

| Emp_ID | Last_Name | First_Name | Cred | Hire_Date |
|--------|-----------|------------|------|-----------|
| 001 | Falk | Susannah | RN | 02/06/2014 |
| 002 | Vargas | Jess | RPT | 12/06/2015 |

a. SELECT Emp_ID, Last_Name, First_Name, Cred FROM Employees WHERE Cred = 'RN'
b. Emp_ID, Last_Name, First_Name, Cred FROM Employees
c. SELECT Emp_ID, Last_Name, First_Name, Cred FROM Employees WHERE = 'RN'
d. SELECT Emp_ID, Last_Name, First_Name, Cred FROM Employees WHERE Clinic = <> 'RN'

**46. A physician is documenting a patient's progress and writes: "Glucose level has stabilized at 110 to 125." If utilizing the SOAP format for problem-oriented recording, in which part would this notation occur?**

    a. Subjective
    b. Objective
    c. Assessment
    d. Plan

**47. Which type of patient record typically includes a problem list?**

    a. Inpatient care
    b. Emergency care
    c. Ambulatory care
    d. Ambulatory surgical care

**48. In order to fully utilize CDS, much of the information within the EHR must be in the form of**

    a. narrative.
    b. discrete data.
    c. continuous data.
    d. images.

**49. Before institution of a new EHR, the HIM department conducts a series of small-scale cognitive walkthrough usability studies with up to 8 participants who practice with prototypes. While the participants practice with the prototypes, they should**

    a. take notes for later review.
    b. "think aloud" about their experience and thoughts.
    c. avoid talking or taking notes.
    d. video tape the exercises for later review.

**50. A healthcare organization has a software license from a software company for 400 networked computers but has opened a new department with 20 additional computers. The department head has copied the application and is using it on the additional computers without notifying the software company. This is an example of**

    a. fair use.
    b. uninformed use.
    c. misuse.
    d. theft.

**51. If changes in software applications will result in the need for completely different procedures to access patient data, including laboratory reports, which of the following is the best way to convey this information to staff?**

    a. Workshops and demonstrations
    b. Email or paper notices
    c. Posters and printed notices
    d. Discussions in staff meetings

**52. A patient hospitalized in an SNF is undergoing occupational therapy. As part of the calculations for reimbursement for care, the total and type of therapy (individual, concurrent, and group) must be calculated. Based on the figures below, group therapy comprises what percentage of total therapy time?**

| Actual OT minutes | Adjusted for reimbursement |
|---|---|
| Individual: 180 | Individual: 100% = 180 |
| Concurrent:100 | Concurrent: 50% = 50 |
| Group: 80 | Group: 25% = 20 |
| Total: 360 minutes | Total: 250 |

a. 22.2%
b. 28.6%
c. 9.5%
d. 8%

**53. If a healthcare organization has networked PHRs that can be accessed by the individual as well as healthcare providers, the principle of *transparency* refers to which of the following?**

a. Patients should provide consent to the collection of data.
b. Patients should control access to the PHRs and be able to easily access data.
c. Patients are advised of the type of data that can be collected, the purpose, and who has access.
d. Data in the PHR is safeguarded against unauthorized use, deletion, or alterations.

**54. A healthcare organization has switched to just-in-time inventory with barcode scanners used to track supplies and automatic ordering carried out when inventory is low. However, some procedures have had to be postponed because delivery of supplies was delayed, and inventory was depleted. What is the likely solution to this problem?**

a. Change vendors.
b. Increase triggers for reordering.
c. Re-educate staff about the procedures.
d. Stop using just-in-time inventory.

**55. When setting up user accounts, which of the following would be classified as a strong password?**

a. Carolina
b. Ilovemycat
c. 12161980
d. D36&lobx

**56. To reduce overtime costs, eight employees in the HIM department are being switched from a 40-hour, 5-day-a-week schedule to a 12-hour, 3-day-a-week schedule in order to provide uninterrupted coverage in the evening. Management projects that only 75% of the lost hours will need to be replaced with part-time workers because of increased efficiency. How many FTE staff members will be needed to replace lost time?**

a. 0.4 FTE
b. 0.5 FTE
c. 0.6 FTE
d. 0.8 FTE

**57. If the HIM department plans to initiate a quality improvement process, staff members should begin with problem identification by**

    a.  identifying key performance measures.

    b.  creating a flow chart.

    c.  conducting a survey.

    d.  brainstorming problems.

**58. An acute care hospital is planning to change to bar-coded patient ID bracelets to meet National Patient Safety Goals of ensuring 2 different forms of ID and reducing medical error. Which barcode scanner type is likely to be the best choice?**

    a.  Linear

    b.  2-dimensional

    c.  Laser

    d.  There is no essential difference

**59. A well-known actor was admitted to an acute care hospital for a drug overdose. When the HIM director reviewed the audit trail for the patient's EHR, it showed that four members of the staff who were not authorized to access the patient's EHR did so. What initial action should the HIM director take?**

    a.  Notify the staff members to stop accessing the EHR.

    b.  Notify the police of unlawful activity.

    c.  Notify the administration of unauthorized access.

    d.  Notify the Secretary of Health and Human Services.

**60. In the five-stage performance management process of planning, monitoring, developing, rating, and rewarding, the primary process that occurs during the developing stage is**

    a.  recognizing achievements.

    b.  providing feedback.

    c.  providing training to employees.

    d.  carrying out performance evaluations.

**61. Under the Two-Midnight rule of CMS, a patient who is admitted to the hospital as an inpatient but stays less than two midnights is eligible for coverage under Medicare A**

    a.  under no circumstances.

    b.  based on physician's expectation of stay beyond two midnights.

    c.  under all circumstances.

    d.  for heart-related admissions only.

**62. According to the data dictionary below regarding healthcare provider information, how many columns would appear in the corresponding table in the database?**

**Healthcare Provider Information**

| Field Name | Length | Data type |
|---|---|---|
| ID # | 5 | Long integer |
| Last_Name | 24 | Alpha |
| First_Name | 22 | Alpha |
| Middle_Name | 5 | Alpha |
| Cred | 10 | Alpha |
| Cred # | 12 | Long integer |

   a. 3
   b. 6
   c. 12
   d. 18

**63. A patient in respiratory distress was placed on BIPAP without intubation for 16 hours and then removed from BIPAP for 2 hours placed back on BIPAP for 4 hours, removed for 3 hours, and then placed back on BIPAP for an additional 8 hours prior to discontinuation. How would the duration be coded for mechanical ventilation under ICD-10-PCS?**

   a. Less than 24 hours
   b. 24 to 96 hours
   c. Greater than 96 hours
   d. Coding as mechanical ventilation is incorrect

**64. If the ICD-10-PCS code for an imaging study of the left clavicle is BP05ZZZ, what type of contrast was used?**

   a. None
   b. Low osmolar
   c. High osmolar
   d. Other

**65. If doing SWOT analysis to assess proposed changes to the information management system, negative attitudes toward change by staff members would be classified as a(n)**

   a. strength.
   b. weakness.
   c. opportunity.
   d. threat.

**66. Which of the following is the primary advantage of an enterprise-wide information system?**

   a. Cost savings related to hardware and software
   b. Reduced staffing needs to manage the information system
   c. Integration among all departments
   d. Improved monitoring of departments

**67. All of the following are common functions of a chief security officer EXCEPT**

    a.  carrying out strategic planning for security of information system.
    b.  developing a security policy for the information system.
    c.  coordinating training of employees regarding security.
    d.  making decisions about purchase of software and hardware.

**68. States have the right to set eligibility criteria for individuals within federal minimum standards for which program?**

    a.  Medicaid
    b.  Medicare
    c.  TRICARE
    d.  Veteran's Health Administration

**69. If a healthcare provider is unable to determine whether a patient's condition at the time the patient was admitted into care was present on admission (POA), which POA option should be selected?**

    a.  Y
    b.  N
    c.  U
    d.  W

**70. Which of the following is an example of *prospective* utilization management?**

    a.  Insurance company requires preauthorization for surgical procedures.
    b.  Patient's care is moved from ICU to cardiac unit as condition improves.
    c.  Patient's care is reviewed to determine if level of care is appropriate.
    d.  Patient's medical claims are denied.

**71. The acute care hospital has a CPOE with CDS system alerts. All of the following are expected outcomes of this system EXCEPT**

    a.  fewer medication errors.
    b.  increased patient participation in care plan.
    c.  elimination of handwritten orders.
    d.  improved pharmacy response time.

**72. Review of patients' EHRs shows that free text documentation by physicians describing patient conditions appears to be identical on consecutive days and on multiple patients' records. Which of the following is the most likely reason for this finding?**

    a.  Patients' conditions remain unchanged.
    b.  Physicians are copying and pasting text.
    c.  Error occurred in computer processing of text.
    d.  Patients' conditions are all the same.

**73. In the table below in a relational database, what will occur if the "Leisure" committee is discontinued and deleted from the database?**

| Emp_ID | Last_Name | First_Name | Cred | Committee |
|--------|-----------|------------|------|-----------|
| 001 | James | Al | RPT | Health |
| 002 | Logan | Seth | RN | Telecom. |
| 003 | Roos | Linda | RN | Leisure |
| 004 | Davidson | Estella | LVN | Telecom. |

a. Linda Roos will be deleted from the database.
b. the entire "Committee" column will be deleted.
c. the "Leisure" field will be replaced by a blank field.
d. the entire table will be deleted of data.

**74. A newer version of the software currently running the EHR has been issued. What type of testing is usually indicated when a new version of software is issued and will be uploaded into the system?**

a. White-box testing
b. Regression testing
c. Non-regression testing
d. Usability testing

**75. In order to submit immunization data electronically to an immunization registry, the organization must first have**

a. VPN.
b. CEHRT.
c. EHR.
d. MAN.

**76. During registration, a patient must sign an *assignment of benefits* form so that**

a. the patient can receive reimbursement for claims.
b. the provider is prohibited from releasing information about the patient.
c. the provider can have access to the healthcare record.
d. the provider can bill the insurance companies.

**77. Under ICD-10-CM, external cause code reporting**

a. may be required by some states or payers.
b. is mandatory.
c. is always voluntary.
d. is never done.

**78. Which of the following was introduced by The Joint Commission (TJC) as part of the accreditation process to integrate outcomes data and performance measurement data?**

a. DEEDS
b. HEDIS
c. ORYX
d. NHIN

**79. During a recent outbreak of SARS, 86 patients were hospitalized with severe complications and 18 patients died in a 30-day period in which 26 patients died of other causes as well. What is the case fatality rate, rounded to the nearest whole number?**

a. 21%
b. 30%
c. 41%
d. 51%

**80. Hospitals may receive Medicare outlier payments for which of the following?**

a. Patient care cases involving clinical trials
b. Patient care cases with exceptionally high cost
c. Patient care cases with no supplementary insurance coverage
d. Patient care cases that involve rare diseases

**81. County Hospital has received a court order requesting documents from a patient's EHR for an attorney representing the patient in a negligence claim. The attorney for the hospital has also requested a copy of the records. The records can be presented in various formats. All of the following are correct about the legal requirements for producing records EXCEPT**

a. only records specifically requested should be provided.
b. records must be presented in exactly the same format to both attorneys.
c. records must be presented in PDF format.
d. all records, including those not specifically asked for, should be provided.

**82. County hospital is reviewing the actual ALOS of 10 patients hospitalized for treatment of ischemic strokes and discharged in a one-week period and comparing results to the MS-DRG GLOS/ALOS to determine which MS-DRG-associated actual ALOS most negatively affects the profit margin. Based on the actual ALOS, for which MS-DRG classification(s) should targeted efforts be made to decrease actual ALOS?**

| MS-DRG | Title | Weight | GLOS | ALOS | Actual ALOS |
|---|---|---|---|---|---|
| 61 | Acute ischemic stroke w thrombolytic w MCC | 2.6877 | 5.4 | 7.1 | 1) 9 2) 7 3) 10 |
| 62 | Acute ischemic stroke w thrombolytic w CC | 1.8906 | 3.9 | 4.6 | 4) 4 5) 3 6) 5 |
| 63 | Acute ischemic stroke w thrombolytic w o CC/MCC | 1.5217 | 2.9 | 3.2 | 7) 4 8) 2 9) 4 10) 2 |

a. 61
b. 62
c. 63
d. 61 and 63

**83. When beginning the design of workload distribution for a distributed database, the initial step should be to analyze**

a. potential outcomes.
b. data access requirements.
c. system and data storage requirements.
d. costs associated with the project.

**84. If a patient is admitted to an acute care hospital on September 6 and discharged on September 18, when does the Medicare benefit period end?**

    a.   November 10
    b.   November 13
    c.   November 15
    d.   November 16

**85. Following a Medicare qualifying stay in an acute care hospital, a patient may be qualified for additional care in a skilled nursing facility (SNF) after discharge from the acute care hospital if admission to the SNF occurs within**

    a.   3 days
    b.   10 days
    c.   30 days
    d.   60 days

**86. If a healthcare provider has accepted assignment for services covered under Medicare, this means that the healthcare provider agrees**

    a.   to charge the patient no more than 115% of allowed charge.
    b.   to accept the allowed charge as payment in full.
    c.   to accept Medicare payment as partial reimbursement only.
    d.   to accept 95% of the payment participating providers receive.

**87. The HIM director is reviewing the chargemaster for accuracy and mapping services to CPS/HCPCS codes. Hardcoding is typically used to ensure accurate billing for all of the following EXCEPT**

    a.   room charges.
    b.   laboratory services.
    c.   ECG.
    d.   respiratory therapy.

**88. Although the volume of patients in outpatient services has increased by 20% over the previous year, a review of revenue shows that services typically provided to outpatients have decreased by 12%, resulting in a loss of revenue. The probable reason for this discrepancy is**

    a.   failure to code for services.
    b.   database error.
    c.   change in procedures.
    d.   inaccurate chargemaster.

**89. Prior to a facility carrying out diagnostic studies to be billed to Medicare, the healthcare provider must**

    a.   notify Medicare.
    b.   document medical necessity.
    c.   seek prior authorization.
    d.   verify supplemental insurance.

**90. A healthcare provider has submitted a claim to Medicare under the Outpatient Prospective Payment System (OPPS), and outpatient code edits (OCE) indicate that there is a diagnosis code for vaginal bleeding during the first trimester of pregnancy but the gender selected is male (edit #3, diagnosis and sex conflict). What claim-level disposition should the healthcare provider expect?**

    a. Denial
    b. Suspension
    c. Rejection
    d. Return

**91. The HIM director has been assigned the position of chief compliance officer after a number of fraudulent practices in claims was identified. The first action of the compliance officer should be to**

    a. discipline those carrying out fraudulent practices.
    b. review and reissue written standards of conduct, polices, and procedures.
    c. establish staff training to ensure compliance.
    d. establish a hotline for complaints.

**92. *Upcoding* occurs when a healthcare provider**

    a. assigns a diagnosis or procedure code that will provide a higher return than the appropriate code.
    b. assigning separate codes to procedures that are usually bundled together under one code.
    c. billing twice for the same service to increase revenue.
    d. changes the code from one system (such as ICD-9) to another (such as ICD-10).

**93. The tool by which the National Committee for Quality Assurance (NCQA) compares the quality of patient care provided by different health plans is**

    a. MEPS.
    b. ANSI 835.
    c. HEDIS.
    d. HCUP.

**94. Where in the patient's record would the following information be found?**

    Ambulatory as desired.
    Acetaminophen 100 mg every 6 hours prn pain.
    Bactrim DS 800/160 mg twice daily for 6 days.

    a. Physician's orders
    b. Nursing notes
    c. Physician's progress notes
    d. Medication record

**95. After the nurse has recorded various measures of a patient in a clinic, the physician reviews the record for the patient's age, weight, gender, pulse, and blood pressure before examining the patient. The term used to describe these facts is**

    a. data sets.
    b. data elements.
    c. information.
    d. aggregate data.

**96. Information in the disease index is considered patient-identifiable data because**

    a. patients with rare diseases may be identifiable.
    b. the patient's name is listed with the disease.
    c. all healthcare information is considered patient-identifiable data.
    d. the disease index links to the EHR by ID number.

**97. When setting up a disease registry from existing data, the first step is to**

    a. establish a time frame.
    b. obtain patient authorization.
    c. develop a case definition.
    d. identify costs associated with the registry.

**98. A patient's discharge summary lists medications as:**

    Metoprolol 50 mg twice daily.
    Hydrochlorothiazide 12.5 mg daily.
    Acetaminophen 600 mg every 4 hours as needed for pain.
    Metformin 850 mg daily.

**The diagnostic information includes primary hypertension (ICD-10-CM, I10), supraventricular tachycardia (ICD-10-CM, I47.1) and bilateral primary osteoarthritis of the knee (ICD-10-CM, M17.0. Based on the list of medications, which diagnosis is missing?**

    a. Diabetes mellitus, type 2 (E11)
    b. Heart attack/Myocardial infarction (I21.4)
    c. COPD (491.22)
    d. Viral pneumonia (J12)

**99. If the hospital administration wants to develop a facility-specific cancer registry, which of the following should the HIM director recommend as the best sources for case finding?**

    a. Discharge summary and disease index
    b. Physician index and disease index
    c. MPI and physician index
    d. MPI and disease index

**100. If a patient suffered a severe reaction when administered the wrong drug and the director of risk management needs a complete description of the incident, the best source of information is the**

    a. physician's progress notes.
    b. nurse's progress notes.
    c. incident report.
    d. discharge summary.

**101. If a medical scribe is used to enter documentation into an EHR for an attending physician, the individual who has the most responsibility to ensure that the EHR is complete and accurate is the**

    a. attending physician.
    b. director of HIM.
    c. director of nursing.
    d. medical scribe.

**102. When reviewing orders for medications, the RHIT should be concerned if a physician has written the following order**

 a. 40 units regular insulin SQ.
 b. Amlodipine, 10.0 mg PO.
 c. Metoprolol, 25 mg BID.
 d. Synthroid, 0.112 mcg daily PO.

**103. CMS provides the following E/M guidelines for determining the type of history (Hx) needed to determine the level of service. Assuming that all four elements in a row must be met to meet the criteria for the type of history, how would a visit with a patient be coded as an E/M service if the physician documented the chief complaint, an extended review of systems, and a pertinent past, family, and/or social history?**

| Type of Hx | Chief Complaint | Hx of present illness | Review of systems | Past, family, and/or social Hx |
|---|---|---|---|---|
| Problem focused | Required | Brief | N/A | N/A |
| Expanded problem focused | Required | Brief | Problem pertinent | N/A |
| Detailed | Required | Extended | Extended | Pertinent |
| Comprehensive | Required | Extended | Complete | Complete |

 a. Expanded problem focused
 b. Detailed
 c. Comprehensive
 d. Does not qualify as an E/M service

**104. In the process of transitioning to an EHR and scanning paper documents, the HIM department has decided to contract with a private agency to destroy paper health records that have been stored for over 10 years. Assuming there are no specific state laws to the contrary, which of the following is NOT necessary to include in the contract?**

 a. Destruction method
 b. Time between acquisition and destruction
 c. Inclusive dates of records
 d. Security measures

**105. Which of the following reference terminologies provides a standardized vocabulary for medical conditions?**

 a. TheraDoc
 b. NMMDS
 c. SNOMED CT
 d. NANDA

**106. With ICD-10-CM, which injury extension is used if, after fracturing a wrist and having a cast applied, the patient returns to the emergency department to have the cast removed?**

 a. A
 b. X
 c. S
 d. D

**107. With ICD-10-PCS, which of the following terms is NOT a root operation?**

    a. Anastomosis
    b. Alteration
    c. Fragmentation
    d. Map

**108. As part of denials management, back-end editing is utilized to**

    a. identify patient accounts that may not demonstrate medical necessity.
    b. identify missing or misplaced charges.
    c. assess efficiency of coding professionals.
    d. identify signs of upcoding.

**109. In a health information organizations with multiple sites accessing the same master patient index, the registration clerk at one facility mistakenly pulls up a record from the master patient index (MPI) for a person with a similar name and demographic information when registering a patient for a procedure. This type of error is referred to as a(n)**

    a. overlap.
    b. duplicate.
    c. corruption.
    d. overlay.

**110. If utilizing the unlisted procedure code under CPT coding for an unlisted chemistry procedure (84999), what further submission is required?**

    a. No further submission
    b. Clinical record with diagnosis, test name, and test results
    c. Test name only
    d. Clinical record with diagnosis only

**111. With CPT coding, if both a CPT modifier code and an HCPCS level II modifier code are utilized to describe a surgical procedure, which modifier code should be placed in the first position?**

    a. CPT modifier
    b. HCPCS level II modifier
    c. Position varies depending on the position
    d. Either can be placed in the first position

**112. If a patient underwent a major surgical procedure, such as an aortic aneurysm repair, how many total days are included in the global surgical package under Medicare guidelines?**

    a. No global surgical package for this procedure
    b. 11 days
    c. 92 days
    d. 122 days

113. A patient was scheduled for a bilateral simple complete mastectomy but, following the procedure on the right breast and after an incision was made for the left, the patient developed severe cardiac dysrhythmias that could not be stabilized. The surgery was discontinued, the incision closed, and the patient sent to the cardiac care unit. Possible modifiers include:

> 53, Reduced services
> 52, Discontinued procedure
> 50, Bilateral
> RT, Right side
> LT, Left side

## How would the procedure be coded?

| CPT/HCPCS Code | Description of Procedure |
| --- | --- |
| 19303 | Mastectomy, simple, complete |

   a. 19303-50-53
   b. 19303-50-52
   c. 19303-50-52-53
   d. 19393-53-LT

114. The purpose of the recovery audit contractor (RAC) program is to

   a. improve documentation.
   b. identify Medicare underpayments.
   c. identify improper Medicare payments.
   d. provide data for research.

115. If paper records that need to be maintained are being moved into a new storage space with bookcase units that are 48 inches wide with 6 shelves per unit, and the average record is one-half inch thick, how many shelving units are needed for 10,080 records?

   a. 15
   b. 18
   c. 25
   d. 35

116. The HIM department has used document imaging to archive medical records. Which of the following can be expected of the imaged records?

   a. They can capture discrete data elements.
   b. They can be accessed for decision support.
   c. They are immediately accessible.
   d. They provide access to patient records.

117. Which characteristic of data quality refers to the use of the specific level of detail required for a data element, such as ensuring three decimal spaces for the laboratory test for specific gravity (1.021)?

   a. Data currency
   b. Data definition
   c. Data granularity
   d. Data precision

**118. Under PQRS Measure #46, Medication Reconciliation, this crosscutting measure must be reported for**

    a. all office or outpatient visits for patients of any age regardless of inpatient status.

    b. outpatient visits with patients 18 and older occurring within 30 days of discharge from inpatient facility.

    c. outpatient visits with patients over age 65 occurring within 30 days of discharge from an inpatient facility.

    d. outpatient visits with patients of any age occurring within 30 days of discharge from an inpatient facility.

**119. The Credentialing and Re-credentialing Committee in an organization is usually NOT responsible for verifying**

    a. current licensure/credentialing.

    b. proof of liability insurance.

    c. credit history.

    d. completion of appropriate education.

**120. The HIM department has received a request from an insurance carrier for a large number of different patient records for claims that do not appear to be problematical. The HIM department should**

    a. question the reason for the requests.

    b. send the records as requested.

    c. refuse to send the records.

    d. send only the records that apply to billing.

**121. Which of the following ICD-10-PCS codes indicates a procedure carried out through an open approach?**

    a. 02703DZ

    b. 0U5B4ZZ

    c. 0T9B70Z

    d. 0FT40ZZ

**122. If a patient is severely allergic to penicillin, which of the following codes is most likely to trigger an alarm any time a penicillin drug is ordered when using a controlled terminology that lists ingredients for the CPOE?**

    a. If ORDER = "penicillin" and ALLERGY = "penicillin" then print "Alert!"

    b. If ORDER = {any ingredient of ordered drug} = {any ingredient of allergic drug} then print "Alert!"

    c. If ORDER = ALLERGY then print "Alert!"

    d. If ORDER = "penicillin" and ALLERGY = "amoxicillin" then print "Alert!"

**123. If an adult hospital wants to meet Leapfrog Group's standards for CPOE, what percentage of physician orders must be made with a CPOE system that contains error-prevention software?**

    a. 25%

    b. 50%

    c. 75%

    d. 90%

**124. County Hospital accepts credit card payments and must comply with security controls set by**

    a. PCI DSS.
    b. COBIT.
    c. NIST SP 800.
    d. SPC.2.

**125. For the HHS Office of Civil Rights (OCR) HIPAA audits, the three compliance categories are**

    a. security, access, breach identification.
    b. safety, security, and encryption.
    c. security, privacy, breach notification.
    d. security, disclosure, privacy.

**126. Based on the General Equivalence Mapping below, what conclusion can be made about mapping the ICD-9-CM codes E850.0 and E851 to ICD-10-CM codes?**

| ICD-9-CM | Description | ICD-10-CM | Description | Approx. | No map |
| --- | --- | --- | --- | --- | --- |
| E850.0 | Accidental poisoning by heroin | | | 0 | 1 |
| E851 | Accidental poisoning by barbiturates | | | 0 | 1 |

    a. These codes can each be approximately matched to one ICD-10-CM code.
    b. These codes cannot be mapped to ICD-10-CM codes.
    c. Each code can be directly matched to one ICD-10-CM code.
    d. Data are insufficient to make conclusions about mapping of the codes.

**127. With ICD-10-PCS, if a patient's gastrostomy tube develops a leak and is removed and a new gastrostomy tube placed into the same opening, the root operation utilized for this procedure is**

    a. replacement.
    b. change.
    c. insertion.
    d. revision

**128. When preparing for an external coding audit, all of the following are appropriate actions for the HIM director to take in regard to coder's concerns EXCEPT**

    a. communicate the goals of the process before the audit begins.
    b. advise coders that the outcomes will be used for disciplinary actions.
    c. stress the educational advantage to the external coding audit.
    d. establish performance goals for individual coding professionals.

**129. Which of the following would be classified as a "Never event" that should never occur in a healthcare setting?**

    a. A patient scheduled for a cholangiogram underwent a colonoscopy in error.
    b. A patient developed a surgical site infection following a cholecystectomy.
    c. A patient tripped and fell, fracturing the right femur.
    d. A patient experienced an adverse effect from analgesia.

**130. In terms of filing claims, "bundling" refers to**

a. sending a number of different claims at the same time.
b. including a number of different procedures under one code.
c. separating linked procedures into different codes.
d. including both CPT codes and ICD-10-PCS codes on claims.

**131. Which of the following would require a HCPCS level II code for a CMS claim?**

a. Ambulance service
b. Blood typing
c. Diagnostic screening
d. Cryopreservation, reproductive tissue, ovarian

**132. If an organization wants to file a Medicare claim for durable medical equipment prosthetics, orthotics, or supplies (DMEPOS) for which no code currently exists, which of the following is the appropriate action?**

a. Use a miscellaneous HCPCS code.
b. Send documentation with the claim.
c. Contact the DME MACs PDAC.
d. No claim can be filed.

**133. If a patient had a kidney removed for "renal cell carcinoma," which column on the ICD-10-CM Table of Neoplasms would the RHIT use to identify the correct code?**

a. Malignant primary
b. Malignant secondary
c. Benign
d. Unspecified behavior

**134. A complete NDC consists of 3 different sub-codes: (1) labeler code, (2) product code, and (3)**

a. FDA code.
b. company code.
c. package code.
d. RX norm code.

**135. The primary purpose of the RxNorm dose form below is to**

| Form | Definition & Usage Notes |
| --- | --- |
| Foam | bubbles of gas that are introduced into a liquid |
| Injectable foam | A foam intended to be injected. |
| Oral foam | A foam intended to be administered into the mouth |
| Rectal foam | A foam intended for use in the rectum |

*Source: National Library of Medicine (NLM).*

a. describe the way in which a drug is administered.
b. describe the form in which a drug is presented.
c. suggest the most common uses of a drug.
d. classify drugs into different categories.

**136. Which of the following is a vocabulary that provides a set of identifiers and names for observations, such as laboratory data?**

   a. UMDNS
   b. ICPC
   c. ICF
   d. LOINC

**137. If a database provides an alert when the patient's birthdate entered into a field shows that the patient being admitted for delivery of an infant is four years old, this type of validation is a(n)**

   a. consistency check.
   b. range check.
   c. numeric check.
   d. completeness check.

**138. Which of the following processes ensures that when claims are filed with Medicare and secondary insurers that the primary insurer is identified as well as secondary insurers and the extent of their contributions?**

   a. Coordination of Benefits
   b. Review of Medical Appeals Council
   c. Beneficiary Notices Initiative
   d. Employer Services

**139. In order to receive Meaningful Use payments, an organization must do all of the following EXCEPT**

   a. conduct a risk analysis.
   b. correct security risks that are identified.
   c. document completion of MU requirements.
   d. Attest that PHI is 100% secure.

**140. According to HIPAA's Privacy Rule, which of the following elements can remain in a health record when the record is de-identified?**

   a. Names
   b. Dates (except year) directly related to the individual
   c. Diagnoses
   d. Medical record numbers

**141. In the revenue cycle, "charge capture" refers to**

   a. payment received for charges.
   b. claims submitted for charges.
   c. account closed after receiving payment.
   d. charges converted to billable fees.

**142. Which of the TRICARE programs represents a preferred provider organization (PPO)?**

   a. TRICARE standard
   b. TRICARE Prime
   c. TRICARE Guard and Reserve
   d. TRICARE Extra

**143. The three levels of severity (MCC, CC, Non-CC) in the MS-DRG system are assigned based on**

    a. primary diagnosis.
    b. secondary diagnoses
    c. LOS.
    d. Wage index.

**144. MS-DRG adjustments to base rate are made based on all of the following EXCEPT**

    a. transfer policy (TP).
    b. value based purchasing (VBP).
    c. disproportionate share hospital (DSH).
    d. indirect medical education (IME).

**145. A physician on staff of County Hospital requests copies of his sister's health records following her hospitalization for an MI. Which is the appropriate response?**

    a. Ask the physician to sign a formal request.
    b. Provide access since the physician is on staff.
    c. Report the physician to the ethics committee.
    d. Refuse the request.

**146. A patient is being treated for recent onset of depression (F06.31), associated with uncontrolled hypothyroidism due to atrophy of the thyroid gland (E03.4). The patient has a history of breast cancer 10 years previously, treated with no current evidence of any existing malignancy (Z85). The patient is currently also receiving treatment for long-term essential hypertension (I10). How would these diagnoses be sequenced (first to last)?**

    a. F06.31, E03.4, I10, and Z85
    b. E03.4, F06.31, Z85, and I10
    c. E03.4, F06.31, I10, and Z85
    d. F06.31, E03.4, Z85, and I10

**147. If County Hospital has an average cost per patient day of $2000 and a case mix index (CMI) of 1.10, its adjusted cost per patient day is**

    a. $2200.00.
    b. $2001.10.
    c. $2420.00.
    d. $1818.18.

**148. If a patient has undergone ambulatory surgery and the physician has written "suspected cholelithiasis" "as the first-listed diagnosis on the front sheet of the patient's record, in order to code the first-listed diagnosis correctly, the coding professional should**

    a. review the operative report for the diagnosis.
    b. use "suspected cholelithiasis" as the diagnosis.
    c. refer the matter to a supervisor for resolution.
    d. send a query to the physician regarding the correct diagnosis.

**149. If an RHIT conducting a record analysis notes that a patient's health record is missing the *Consent for Operation and/or Procedures*, the RHIT should**

    a.  send a notice to the physician to obtain the consent.
    b.  take no action as it is unrelated to coding.
    c.  assume the patient was unable to sign.
    d.  notify a supervisor who can address the issue.

**150. Before assigning an APC code to a claim for an outpatient procedure in an ambulatory surgery center, the coding professional must first assign an ICD-10-CM diagnostic code, and a(n)**

    a.  CPT/HCPCS code.
    b.  ICD-10-PCS code.
    c.  NDC.
    d.  point of origin code.

**151. The total charges for a healthcare organization for May are $132,000.00 and net collections are $92,000.00. The organization's average monthly charges are $128,000. What is the A/R ratio, expressed in percentage?**

    a.  31.25%
    b.  71.8%
    c.  14%
    d.  69.6%

**152. If the HIM director is managing a project to upgrade the HIM system, the three project cost management processes the director must carry out are (1) estimating costs, (2) establishing a budget, and (3)**

    a.  conducting reviews.
    b.  maintaining a timeline.
    c.  controlling costs.
    d.  filing reports.

**153. A large hospital has the same coders coding both inpatient and outpatient records, but a coding audit shows there have been increasing numbers of errors in coding over the previous 6 months. The best solution may be to**

    a.  change to coding specialization.
    b.  provide increased training.
    c.  provide incentives for improved performance.
    d.  provide disciplinary action for poor performance.

**154. If a physician at an ambulatory surgery center carries out a procedure normally done only as an inpatient, and the OPPS status indicator for the HCPCS/CPT code is "C," what type of OPPS reimbursement should be expected?**

    a.  Standard reimbursement for procedure
    b.  No reimbursement
    c.  Partial reimbursement (50%)
    d.  Partial reimbursement, equipment and supplies only

**155.** The supervisor of the cardiac care unit and the HIM director are reviewing statistics regarding selected DRG codes for the unit. Based on the number of discharges and the relative weights for each DRG, which code has resulted in the highest reimbursement?

| Diagnostic Related Group Code and Description | Rel. Weight | # Discharges |
|---|---|---|
| 291 – Heart failure and shock w MCC | 1.4822 | 1208 |
| 292 – Heart failure and shock wo MCC | 0.9703 | 2506 |
| 280 – Acute myocardial infarction discharged alive w MCC | 1.6969 | 1846 |
| 281 – Acute myocardial infarction discharged alive w CC | 1.0236 | 1286 |
| 282 – Acute myocardial infarction discharged alive wo CC MCC | 0.7823 | 2078 |
| 283 – Acute myocardial infarction expired w MCC | 0.7824 | 102 |

    a. 291
    b. 292
    c. 280
    d. 282

**156.** If a hospital had 826 discharges over a 30-day period and experienced 32 deaths, including 2 newborns, 4 children, and 3 adults who died within 48 hours of admission, the gross death rate (rounded to one decimal point) for this period is

    a. 3.8%.
    b. 3.6%.
    c. 3.5%.
    d. 3.1%.

**157.** From an ethical perspective, which of the follow principles is operational if the HIM professional releases information about a patient only with proper authorization and for the good of the patient?

    a. Justice
    b. Autonomy
    c. Nonmaleficence
    d. Beneficence

**158.** A potentially compensable event is

    a. an event for which an organization can bill an insurance company.
    b. a claim for which an insurance company has requested information.
    c. an action for which a provider can file a claim for reimbursement.
    d. an incident that can lead to financial loss or legal action.

**159.** According to the physician's notes, an outpatient complained of pain in the right knee. The physician ordered an x-ray of the right knee as well as a complete blood count (CBC), metabolic panel, and chest x-ray. The CBC showed an elevated white count (10,000) and the metabolic panel showed a slightly elevated glucose (106). How should the coding professional code the diagnosis/diagnoses?

    a. Code M25.561, Pain in right knee only
    b. Code M25.561, Pain in right knee, and query physician regarding further diagnoses
    c. Code M25.561, Pain in right knee; and A49.9 bacterial infection, unspecified
    d. Code M25.561, Pain in right knee; A49.9 bacterial infection, unspecified; and Z13.1 encounter for screening for diabetes

**160.** County hospital has experienced a recent increase in medical-necessity denials from Medicare, and the different levels of appeals and costs involved have negatively impacted the return on investment. If the hospital wants to determine the cause of the denials and take steps to remedy the situation, the best place to begin is by

a. assessing claims data.
b. educating physicians.
c. assessing denials data.
d. educating coding professionals.

**161.** In a recent 30-day period, 46 infants were discharged from the NICU. During that time, an outbreak of *Enterobacteriaceae* occurred with 8 infants infected. What is the infection rate for this 30-day period (rounded to one decimal point)?

a. 16.8%
b. 17.4%
c. 26.6%
d. 38.0%

**162.** If an outpatient radiological procedure with contrast resulted in a lump-sum payment for both the technical component of the procedure and the professional component, this type of payment is referred to as

a. prospective.
b. fee-for-service.
c. bundled.
d. global.

**163.** According to NHIN, the three dimensions of infrastructure needed for HIM systems are (1) personal health dimension, (2) healthcare provider dimension, and (3)

a. equipment/supplies dimension.
b. education dimension.
c. population health dimension.
d. core data elements dimension.

**164.** If a patient of a home health agency required only 4 visits in a 60-day period, what impact will this have on Medicare reimbursement?

a. No impact
b. Low-utilization payment adjustment (LUPA)
c. Partial episode payment (PEP)
d. Denial of claim

**165.** If a patient was admitted to the hospital with severe headache but the physician failed to order a head CT and discharged the patient, who subsequently died with a subdural hemorrhage, the type of negligence that could be charged is

a. nonfeasance.
b. malfeasance.
c. misfeasance.
d. defeasance.

# Answer Key and Explanations

**1. A:** The Medicare Outpatient Code Editor (OCE) conducts the following types of edits:

Coding: Ensures claim does not include inpatient only procedures and that codes are valid and there are no age or gender conflicts.

Coverage: Ensures claims are for covered procedures.

Clinical: Ensures demographic information is correct.

Claims: Ensures dates, units of service and observations are appropriate.

**2. B:** When calculating the fetal death rate for the hospital, all fetal deaths occurring at or after 20 weeks' gestation or weight of equal to or greater than 501 g should be included in the calculation. Early fetal deaths occurring prior to 20 weeks' gestation or with a weight of 500 g or less are not counted in the fetal death rate. Fetal deaths are classified by gestation and weight:

Early: under 20 weeks and under 500 g.

Intermediate: 20-28 weeks or more and weight of 501 to 1000 g.

Late: 28 weeks or more and weight over 1000 g.

To calculate fetal death rate:

$$\frac{\text{Total \# intermediate and late fetal deaths}}{[\text{Total \# live births}] + [\text{total \# intermediate and late fetal deaths}]}$$

**3. D:** If an insurer, such as Blue Cross/Blue Shield, denies a claim, an internal appeal (carried out by the insurance company) must be submitted within 180 days of the denial. The insurance company must complete the appeals process and render a decision within 30 days for future services and 60 days for services already received. If the insurer continues to deny the claim, the claimant has 60 days after notification of the denial to request an external review carried out by a third party.

**4. C:** A computer worm is a program that is able to duplicate itself (rather than attaching to another program) and spreads throughout a system. A computer virus is a program that reproduces itself and then attaches to a program in order to corrupt data. A Trojan horse allows unauthorized access to a computer in order to gain information or to send emails. A rootkit is a program that gains access to a computer's operating system in order to modify it.

**5. B:** The out-of-pocket cost the patient will incur is $117.60. Since Medicare pays only 80% of the UCR charge ($240×.80), Medicare normally pays $192 for the visit. However, because the physician is non-participating, and has not accepted assignment the physician receives only 95% of the usual payment ($192×.95) or $182.40 ($300 − $182.40 = $117.60).

**6. D:**

| Patient's financial responsibilities | |
|---|---|
| Deductible | $150 annually |
| Office visits (OV) | $20 copayment |
| Laboratory tests | $5 copayment per lab test |
| CT, MRI, PET scan | $25 copayment per test |
| X-ray | $10 copayment per order |
| ED visit | $100 copayment |
| **Patient's medical expenses** | | | |

| Service | Unit cost | Unit # | Total cost |
|---|---|---|---|
| Office visits (OV) | $110.00 | 8 | $880.00 |
| Laboratory tests | Varies | 10 | $285.00 |
| MRI | $1500.00 | 1 | $1500.00 |
| ED visit | $600.00 | 1 | $600.00 |
| X-ray | $120.00 | 1 | $120.00 |
| **TOTAL** | | | $3385.00 |

Based on the patient's financial responsibility, the patient would need to pay a total of $495.00:

$$= \text{deductible} + (\text{OV} \times 8) + (\text{Lab} \times 10) + (\text{MRI}) + (\text{ED}) + (\text{x-ray})$$
$$= \$150 + \$160 + \$50 + \$25 + \$100 + \$10$$
$$= \$495$$

**7. C:** If a healthcare organization wants a classification system to quantify levels of functioning, disability, and health, the best option is ICF (International Classification of Functioning, Disability, and Health). There are 4 code components to the ICF in 2 parts:

Part I: Functioning and Disability: Body Structure and Body Function.

Part II: Contextual Factors: Activities and Participation and Environmental Factors.

Impairment is quantified from 0 (none) to 4 (complete) with code 8 indicating "not specified" and 9 "not applicable."

**8. A:** If a patient is being treated specifically with immunotherapy (or chemotherapy or radiation therapy) for a malignancy, the therapy is listed as the principle diagnosis (Z51.2), followed by the condition to which the therapy applies, multiple myeloma (C90.00). Other chronic conditions are then listed, such as SVT (I46.1). Codes sequence is: Z51.12, C90.00, and I46.1.

**9. B:** When calculating the readmission adjustment factor (RAF) for MS-DRG base rate, if the operating DRG is $5040 and the RAF is 0.9990 less 1.0, the adjustment to the base rate is (-$5.04) to bring the base rate to $5034.96. Calculations are made based on whether the RAF is more or less than 1:

$$0.0990 - 1.0 = (-0.0010)$$

$$\$5040 \times (-0.0010) = (-\$5.04)$$

Under provisions of the Affordable Care Act, payments to IPPS hospitals are reduced if they have excess readmissions.

**10. D:** When billing for dental claims, the CDT (Current Dental Terminology), coding system is utilized. CDT was developed by the American Dental Association (ADA). The code contains 12 categories of service, covering different types of dental services (such a preventive, orthodontics, and periodontics) with code series ranging from D0100-D9999. Coding is arranged according to procedure category, procedural subcategory, code number, and nomenclature.

**11. D:** In HCPSC level II codes, J codes are used for drugs that are not administered orally, such as chemotherapy drugs and inhalational drugs. A codes are used for transportation services, such as ground and air ambulance. D codes are used for dental procedures and comprise a CDT code set copyrighted by the American Dental Association (ADA). E codes are used for durable medical equipment, such as bathtub wall rail and oxygen equipment and supplies.

**12. C:** Forms control is a process in which specific forms are created for specific purposes and then maintained by medical records departments. Usually committees meet to design forms, such as admission, history and physical, and nursing note, which will be used by a facility. While forms are not completely standardized, they must contain certain information, so forms from one facility to another are often similar. The documents are contained in charts (paper or electronic) and are examined for completeness before being filed or stored.

**13. A:** The purpose of a clinical pertinence review is to ensure documentation is correct. The clinical pertinence review is done retrospectively, usually by pulling a percentage of each physician's charts or a percentage from each department. Forms usually evaluated for completion include the history and physical, family history, and discharge summary. If handwritten notes are included, they are evaluated for legibility. Proper use of abbreviations and symbols is evaluated. Laboratory findings are assessed as well as follow-up for abnormal results.

**14. B:** If one procedure always involves 5 separate charges, but errors in coding for the charges frequently result in omission of one or two charges, the best solution may be to utilize a charge explosion code. With this type of coding, the healthcare provider has to only enter one code for the procedure. This code is linked to the five different charges so that when the procedure code is selected, it pulls up all of the charges.

**15. D:** If a patient was hospitalized in the psychiatric unit for 60 days following a suicide attempt and the insurance company has requested a copy of the psychiatrist's psychotherapy notes, the correct response is to decline to send a copy of the notes. Psychotherapy notes are not considered part of the EHR by HIPAA and do not contain information needed for claims. Psychotherapy notes can be released by court order or with express authorization of the patient.

**16. C:** The *guarantor* of an account is the person who is responsible for paying bills not paid for by insurance. In some cases, this may be the person for whom the account is established, but in other cases, it may be a parent or other individual. If the patient is not the guarantor of his/her account, then the name, address, and contact information (phone number, email address) of the guarantor must be recorded for billing purposes.

**17. A:** Preparation for an accreditation survey by The Joint Commission (TJC) should be an ongoing process that an organization is involved in every day rather than just as preparation for reviews. TJC does a complete survey on a minimum 3-year cycle, but TJC issues yearly standards updates, and organizations accredited by TJC are expected to meet these standards. The Joint Commission accredits acute care, ambulatory care, and rehabilitation organizations as well as hospices and home health agencies.

**18. B:** The primary difference between licensed beds in a facility and the bed count is that the bed count is the number of beds that are ready for patients and staffed, whether or not they are filled with patients. The licensed bed count is the number of beds that have been approved for the facility by the state. If the census drops, facilities often close sections to decrease the bed count, but if the bed count is consistently lower than the licensed beds, this may indicate there is insufficient need for beds.

**19. B:** When calculating the average length of day based on discharges in a 7-day period, the calculation is based on the number of discharges and the length of stay of each person discharged:

Total lengths of stay divided by total number of discharges = average length of stay

$$15 \times 4 = 60, \quad 1 \times 20 = 20, \quad 4 \times 2 = 8, \quad 5 \times 1 = 5, \quad 1 \times 7 = 7$$

$$60 + 20 + 8 + 5 + 7 = 100 \text{ total}$$

$$100 \div 25 = 4 \text{ average length of stay in the oncology unit}$$

The average length of stay can be calculated based on any designated period. Weekly time ALOS may be calculated to evaluate progress at decreasing LOS while annual ALOS may be calculated for year-end reports.

**20. D:** If a patient is treated in the emergency department for 2 hours and then kept for observation in a special unit adjacent to the emergency department for 36 hours following a concussion and episodes of confusion, the patient is classified as an outpatient for the entire stay. Patients may be kept as outpatients for observation for up to 48 hours, regardless of where in the facility they are maintained. If they must remain after this period of time, they are admitted as inpatients.

**21. A:** Based on the data in the table regarding average length of stay by department over a 6-month period, there has been almost no change. The ALOS varied from a low of 4.8 (March) to a high of 5.1 (February) with January and June both averaging 4.9. As is common, mental health patients tend to have higher ALOS than patients in other departments, and patients in OBGYN tend to have the shortest ALOS.

**22. C:** An RN is not classified as a clinical allied health professional. The RN, including NPs and CRNAs and other nursing specialties, is a direct care provider along with MDs, LVNs/LPNs, and PAs. Clinical allied health professionals include a wide range of health professionals who provide services to patients, including OTs, RTs, PTs, clinical laboratory technicians, pharmacists, dietitians, audiologists, speech pathologists, phlebotomists, medical assistants, home health aides, and social workers.

**23. C:** Because outpatients do not generally stay for prolonged periods, the size of an outpatient facility, such as a physical therapy center, is determined by the visits/encounters per day, so size is efficiency-based. Thus, a facility that serves 200 patients per day is twice the size of one that serves 100 patients per day, regardless of the physical size of the facility or the number of beds or other pieces of equipment available.

**24. D:** In order to comply with accreditation standards of TJC, a complete history and appropriate physical examination must be completed for an inpatient by a qualified healthcare provider within 24 hours after admission to an acute care facility. Specialists, such as podiatrists, may complete the part of the history and physical exam that relate to their specialty. The history and physical examination are critical components needed for a diagnosis and treatment of the patient.

**25. B:** PHI refers to protected health information. PHI is information that is created or received by a healthcare provider and that may be recorded in any form (written, visual, electronic, or oral). PHI may cover the health information in the past as well as in the present and in the anticipated future. PHI covers both mental and physical conditions and any treatment provided for these conditions. The HIPAA Privacy Rule covers health information in any form but the HIPAA Security Rule is limited to EPHI (electronic).

**26. D:** The American College of Surgeons first developed a health initiative that required hospitals to keep records of care and treatment in the year 1918. Before 1918, it was the physician's responsibility to keep records, and there were no established standards for what the records should include or how long they should be retained. Early records usually included brief nursing notes but often lacked such important information as diagnosis, history, and physical examination.

**27. D:** Under HIPAA's Privacy Rule, *consent* is for use of PHI (not for treatment as with *informed* consent). Consent means that the healthcare providers can use PHI. Patients are usually given a copy of the privacy policy for the healthcare provider. Signing this form indicates that the person has given permission for the use of the PHI covered by the privacy policy. PHI may be used for some purposes without authorization, including use to provide treatment and disclosure of information for insurance claims.

**28. A:** A physical safeguard of the security standards in HIPAA includes restricted access to EPHI as well as keeping off-site computer backups to prevent loss of records. Other types of safeguards include administrative (security training, delegation of security response) and technical (authentication controls, encryption/decryption). There are a number of standards for each category of safeguards. In addition, the Security Rule includes implementation specifications, which are either required or addressable (not optional). For example, a security management process is required and security awareness and training is addressable.

**29. B:** In the relational database, the foreign keys are Customer ID# and Product # as these link to the primary keys in table 1 (ID #) and table 3 (Product #). In a relational database, data are organized into tables that are related, based on logical groupings. The primary key is one that provides a unique identifier while the foreign key is the common field that links tables and is not a primary key.

**30. A:** In ASCII (American Standard Code for Information Interchange), bytes with a value of 32 to 126 are used to represent numbers, letters, and punctuation (the letter A represents the number 65). Bytes from 1 to 31 control the flow of information in the computer (the number 2, for example, represents the start of text). Higher values, 127 to 257 are used for extended characters and symbols. ASCII standardized text bytes in 1963.

**31. C:** A database is essentially a collection of data. The smallest unit of text data is the character, which may be letters, numbers, spaces, or punctuation marks. Data are divided into defined logical units by fields (numeric, text, dates). Groups of fields the comprise records, which are about a specific thing. For example, database may contain many records showing individual's names and addresses. Records are grouped into tables, which can then be linked.

**32. C:** Images, such as MRI images, CT images, and x-rays are captured, stored, printed, and distributed according to DICOM (Digital Imaging and Communication in Medicine) standards. DICOM allows various types of hardware (such as scanners, servers, printers, and computer workstations) produced by different manufacturers to integrate and form a picture archiving and communication system (PACS). The first standard was released in 1985 and second, which was improved, in 1988, but it wasn't referred to as DICOM until the third version in 1993.

**33. B:** Payment floor refers to the time period when Medicare/insurance companies delay sending reimbursement after adjudication. A *floor* refers to the minimum time a claim is held and a *ceiling* to the maximum. Medicare has a 28-day payment floor for paper claims and a 13-day payment floor for electronic claims, which are less time-intensive to adjudicate. Therefore, it is the advantage of healthcare organizations to utilize electronic billing.

**34. D:** CCOM (Clinical Context Object Workgroup) is a subset of HL7. With an electronic health record that utilizes software applications from different vendors, the CCOM standards allow the user to log in one time for all of the applications. One logged in, as the user switches applications, the person is automatically logged in to the new application and the necessary information (patient ID, provider, and visit) is carried over through context management. Setting up CCOM is quite complex and requires special servers.

**35. B:** According to the Payback on Investment graph, payback occurred at year 2 when the cumulative costs reached $370,000 and the cumulative benefits reached the same number. The organization did not experience the immediate payback that it expected although the benefits have steadily improved and maintenance costs are slowing. Beyond the point where the lines cross (benefits – costs = 0), the organization shows profit. A one-year payback period is often expected of organizations, but long-term goals should also be considered.

**36. C:** Health insurance claims utilize aggregate data and are not primary health records but secondary. Information, such as diagnosis, treatment, and procedures, is taken from the primary record of the patient for health insurance claims and coded in order to bill for payment. Other secondary health records include the mater patient index (MPI), which contains key identifying information about clients so that duplicate records are avoided, and any aggregate data collected for analysis, such as data regarding LOS.

**37. A:** With the ICD-10-PCS procedure code, the letters that are not used are I and O because they could be confused with the numbers one (1) and zero (0). The ICD-10-PCS code requires 7 digits and is a combination of letters (not case sensitive) and numbers. For example, the following code 0FB03ZX is code for "Excision of liver, percutaneous approach, diagnostic." ICD-10-PCS codes do not contain decimals although ICD-10-CM diagnoses codes contain 3 to 7 digits with the first always alpha and the second numeric with a decimal after the third digit.

**38. D:** The Resident-Assessment Instrument (RAI) is required by CMS for long-term care facilities. RAI contains the Minimum Data Set (MDS), the Care Area Assessment (CAA) and a guide to utilization. MDS is used to assess clinical and functional status. CAA is then utilized to make decisions about any problems identified and to develop a plan of care, implement the plan and evaluate outcomes. RAI promotes individualized care and improved communication among staff members.

**39. B:** According to AHIMA's minimum retention periods, adult health records should be retained for 10 years following the last encounter. CMS requires that health records be retained for minimum time periods as well although some states may require longer retention, so it's important to check both federal and state laws. Because many records are now stored digitally, they may be saved permanently because of ease of storage and minimal costs to retain them.

**40. C:** A secondary purpose of an electronic health records is one that does not involve the direct care of the patient or an encounter between a healthcare provider and a patient. Secondary purposes relate to education, litigation, regulation, policymaking, and research. An example of a secondary purpose is when the health record serves as evidence in litigation, such as when a patient sues for malpractice. Other secondary purposes include to carry out research about clinical practices, outcomes, populations, and products; to allocate resources' to educate healthcare professionals; and to provide information for presentations.

**41. A:** If a rash on a patient's torso is described by different healthcare providers as "macular," "papular," "measles-like," "red," "raised," and "allergic," the quality characteristics of data quality management that this violates is data consistency because the information provided is not reliable. The actual appearance of the rash is not evident from the various descriptions. These various descriptions may interfere with diagnosis and treatment and make coding for reimbursement difficult. Some inconsistencies, such as change in diagnosis over time, may legitimately occur.

**42. A:** The system of numbering for charts used when a patient is assigned a number on a first admission to a hospital and is assigned the same number with each subsequent admission is unit numbering. Unit numbering makes accessing previous records of a patient easier than other number types, such as serial numbering in which one patient could end up with multiple charts with different numbers. With serial-unit numbering, serial numbers are applied at each admission and previous records are upgraded to the new number. Family numbering is sometimes used to connect family records, such children of one set of parents.

**43. D:** A description of anesthesia is not found in a diagnostic report but rather in the anesthesia report that is completed by the anesthesiologist. Diagnostic reports may contain many different types of laboratory reports, such as CBC and BUN, from blood specimens or other body fluids (urine, sputum, cerebrospinal fluid, sperm, and vaginal discharge). Diagnostic reports can also include microscopic analysis of tissue samples and monitors and tracings, such as the electrocardiogram and electroencephalogram, which show body functions.

**44. D:** The Security Management Process for HIPAA's Security Management Standard begins with (1) risk analysis. Potential risks to security should be identified and evaluated in terms of the likelihood of occurrence and the degree of seriousness. Other implementations include (2) risk management, which requires decisions regarding how to manage security risks and developing strategies to protect data; (3) sanction policy, which should outline sanctions and/or disciplinary actions for those who fail to maintain security standards; and (4) information systems activity review, which requires audit and review of records to determine if EPHI has been secure.

**45. A:**

**Employees**

| Emp_ID | Last_Name | First_Name | Cred | Hire_Date |
| --- | --- | --- | --- | --- |
| 001 | Falk | Susannah | RN | 02/06/2014 |
| 002 | Vargas | Jess | RPT | 12/06/2015 |

If using SQL to query a relational database with the headings as in the table above, the correct query for a list of the names of RNs only, including their employee IDs is:

SELECT Emp_ID, Last_Name, First_Name, Cred FROM Employees

WHERE Cred = 'RN'

**46. C:** If utilizing the SOAP format for problem-oriented recording, the physician statement "Glucose level has stabilized at 110 to 125" would be entered in the assessment portion of the notes. SOAP notes include assessment data, a list of patient problems, numbered sequentially, and a structured format for documenting. The SOAP format:

Subjective: Patient's statement or description of problem.

Objective: Clinical findings and observations.

Assessment: Conclusions based on subjective and objective findings.

Plan: Plan of action to solve or manage problem.

**47. C:** Ambulatory care records typically contain a problem list to help with the management of ongoing problems. Problem lists are utilized in situations where a patient is likely to be followed for an extended period of time, such as in clinics, outpatient facilities, or physician's office. Problems are typically numbered and the date noted when they are added to the list. Typically, a problem list includes current health problems and significant past conditions, injuries, surgeries, or illnesses. The date should be noted when a problem is resolved.

**48. B:** In order to fully utilize CDS, much of the information within the EHR must be in for form of discrete data, which comprise raw facts and figures, such as lab values, dates, scores, and dosages. With discrete data, the CDS application can help healthcare providers to make decisions if the data are adequate, and reports and charts are easy to generate. The need for discrete data is one of the reasons that EHRs have less narrative than traditional paper charts.

**49. B:** If the HIM department is conducting a series of small-scale cognitive walkthrough usability studies with up to 8 participants, while the participants practice, they should talk aloud (referred to as "think aloud") about their experiences, feelings, and concerns. Observers take notes of what the participants are saying, and these notes are later reviewed to determine areas of concern. These types of studies are especially valuable to determine how much difficulty is involved in the use of hardware/software and how much training will be necessary prior to implementation.

**50. D:** If a healthcare organization has a software license from a software company for 400 networked computers but has opened a new department with 20 additional computers and the department head has copied the application and is using it on the additional computers without notifying the software company, this is an example of theft. Proprietary software developed and licensed by a company is protected by patent and/or copyright and cannot be used beyond the terms of the contract and license.

**51. A:** If changes in software applications will result in the need for completely different procedures to access patient data, including laboratory reports, the best way to convey this information to staff is through workshops and demonstrations. This should be carried out before implementation so that the staff is prepared for the changes. Written guidelines, such as in handbooks or posters, should also be available for staff members to refer to if the need arises.

**52. D:** Group therapy comprises 8% of the total therapy time.

| Actual OT minutes | Adjusted for reimbursement |
|---|---|
| Individual: 180 | Individual: 100% = 180 |
| Concurrent: 100 | Concurrent: 50% = 50 |
| Group: 80 | Group: 25% = 20 |
| Total: 360 minutes | Total: 250 |

The full time is reported for individual therapy but only 50% for concurrent and 25% for group therapy because concurrent therapy and group therapy requires less time and effort on the part of the therapist.

$$180 + 50 + 20 = 250$$

$$\frac{20}{250} = 0.08 \rightarrow 8\%$$

Group therapy should not exceed 25% of total therapy time. If it does, then adjusted minutes must be calculated, resulting in lower reimbursement.

**53. C:** If a healthcare organization has networked PHRs that can be accessed by the individual as well as healthcare providers, the principle of *transparency* refers to patients being advised of the type of data that can be collected, the purpose, and who has access. Other principles include the patients' rights to consent to the collection of data and privacy/security to ensure that data are safeguarded. Patients should have control over their PRHs, and quality is demonstrated through accurate up-to-date information. Oversight and trouble-shooting should be readily available.

**54. B:** If a healthcare organization has switched to just-in-time inventory with barcode scanners used to track supplies and automatic ordering carried out when inventory is low, but some procedures have had to be postponed because delivery of supplies was delayed, the likely solution to this problem is to increase triggers for reordering. This scenario suggests that the inventory levels are set too low. Careful review should be carried out to determine what levels need to be adjusted. Just-in-time inventory often results in the use of fewer vendors but considerable cost savings.

**55. D:** When setting up user accounts, D36&lobx would be classified as a strong password because it is 8 characters in length and is a combination of uppercase letters, lower case letters, numbers, and symbols. The user should avoid names (such as Carolina, of family members, friends, or animals) or phrases (such as Ilovemycat). Dates should be avoided (such as wedding anniversaries and birthdates 12161980 [12-16-1980]) because they are commonly used and easy to guess.

**56. C:** If 8 employees in the HIM department are switching from a 40-hour, 5-day-a-week schedule to a 12-hour, 3-day-a-week schedule in order to provide uninterrupted coverage in the evening, and management projects that only 75% of the lost hours will need to be replaced with part-time workers because of increased efficiency, 0.6 FTE staff members will be needed to replace lost time. Calculations:

$$(\text{number of employees}) \times (\text{number of lost hours}) = 8 \times 4 = 32$$

$$32 \times 0.75\% = 24$$

$$\frac{24}{40} = 0.6 \text{ FTE needed}$$

**57. A:** If the HIM department plans to initiate a quality improvement process, staff members should begin with problem identification by identifying key performance measures, such as the number of records processed per hour or the time needed to respond to a service call. This may entail measuring current performance in order to arrive at realistic measures. Then, a flow chart should be created showing the current process and brainstorming carried out to identify problems with the process. Regulatory requirements should be investigated, and performance compared with benchmark standards. Surveys may be conducted for input and problems prioritized.

**58. B:** If an acute care hospital is planning to change to bar-coded patient ID bracelets to meet National Patient Safety Goals of ensuring 2 different forms of ID and reducing medical error, the barcode scanner type that is likely to be the best choice is the 2-dimensional scanner type. While linear and laser barcode scanner types can only be scanned in one direction—horizontally and lined up with barcode—the 2 dimensional scanner type can be scanned from any direction, saving time and allowing easier scanning without disturbing the patient.

**59. D:** If an audit trail showed that four members of the staff who were not authorized to access a famous actor's EHR did so, the initial action should be to notify the administration so that action can be taken against the staff members unless mitigating circumstances apply (such as a request by a physician to check information on an EHR). In many cases, unauthorized access of EHRs is grounds for dismissal. Other notifications are required (patient, HHS), and some states have requirements in addition to federal requirements.

**60. C:** In the five-stage performance management process, the primary process that occurs during the developing stage is providing training to employees. The five-stage process is as follows:

Planning: Define goals and decide how to apply performance standards.

Monitoring: Monitor performance standards.

Developing: Train employees.

Rating: Conduct performance evaluations to determine if procedures are being carried out appropriately.

Rewarding: Recognize compliance and excellence.

**61. B:** Under the Two-Midnight rule of CMS, a patient who is admitted to the hospital as an inpatient but stays less that two midnights is eligible for coverage under Medicare A based on the physician's expectation that the patient's condition is such that a stay of beyond two midnights is warranted. Generally, the Two-Midnight rule states that patient's with stays of less than two midnights are billed as outpatients under Medicare B and those of more than two midnights as inpatients under Medicare A.

**62. B:** According to the data dictionary regarding healthcare provider information, 6 columns would appear in the corresponding table in the database with the fields in the order listed in the data dictionary:

| ID # | Last_Name | First_Name | Middle_Name | Cred | Cred # |
|------|-----------|------------|-------------|------|--------|
| 010 | Wiley | Jasper | Monroe | MD | 18888 |
| 066 | Walters | Sarah | Faye | MD | 17722 |
| 103 | Aiken | Jennifer | Marie | RN | 41759 |

**63. D:** Regardless of the duration of BIPAP without intubation, coding as mechanical ventilation is incorrect because BIPAP without intubation is coded as "assistance with respiratory ventilation" rather than "respiratory ventilation," which means that respirations are completely under control of the ventilation equipment. The duration of all types of respiratory ventilation should be carefully calculated and the exact hours noted when ventilation is started and discontinued. Calculations are based on hours and not days.

**64. A:** If the ICD-10-PCS code for an imaging study of the right clavicle is BP05ZZZ, then no contrast was used. Code contains 7 characters:

1. Section (imaging): B
2. Body system (non-axial upper bones): P
3. Root type (radiography, plain): 0
4. Body part: left clavicle: 5
5. Contrast (none): Z
6. Qualifier (none): Z
7. Qualifier (none): Z

**65. D:** If doing SWOT (strength, weakness, opportunity, threat) analysis to assess proposed changes to the information management system, negative attitudes toward change by staff members would be classified as a threat. Threats and weaknesses should receive as much or more consideration than strengths and opportunities. In the planning process, attitudes are often overlooked, but positive attitudes toward proposed changes are often critical to success. For this reason, staff members should be engaged in planning and implementation at all stages in the change process.

**66. C:** The primary advantage of an enterprise-wide information system is integration among all departments because the system manages all aspects of the healthcare business. This integration improves the ability to gather and analyze data and to make decisions. In some cases, enterprise-wide information systems may result in cost savings, but the initial outlay for the system can be costly so increased efficiency is usually the primary benefit.

**67. D:** The chief security officer is not generally responsible for making decisions about the purchase of hardware and software because the chief security officer's primary concern is to ensure that data are secure. Among the common functions of the chief security officer are carrying out strategic planning for the security of the information system, developing a security policy, and coordinating training of employees. The chief security officer should also manage any confidentiality agreements, such as with contractors, and should monitor audit trails and conduct risk assessment of enterprise systems.

**68. A:** States have the right to set eligibility criteria for individuals within federal minimum standards for Medicaid. States must cover some groups, such as low-income families with children, children below age 6, and pregnant women with family income at or below 133% of the Federal

Poverty Level. States may, if they choose, cover additional groups through expanded coverage. Laws regarding Medicaid include estate recovery, meaning that the state can recover some benefits paid to an individual from the individual's estate after the person dies.

**69. D:** If a healthcare provider is unable to determine whether a patient's condition at the time the patient was admitted into care was present on admission (POA), the POA option that should be selected is "W." This choice is considered by CMS as a "Y" (yes) for payment purposes. If the conditions are present, the POA option is "Y," and if it is not present, "N." The option "U" is used if documentation is not adequate to determine whether or not the condition was POA. "U" is considered by CMS as an "N" for payment purposes.

**70. A:** An example of prospective utilization management is when an insurance company requires preauthorization for surgical procedures. This allows the company to review the case and determine if the medical services proposed are appropriate. Utilization may also be done concurrently, such as when a patient's level of care is evaluated and the patient is moved from ICU to a cardiac unit as condition improves. Retrospective utilization management is carried out when records are reviewed after medical services are provided, such as when medical claims are denied.

**71. B:** If an acute care hospital has a CPOE with CDS system alerts, it is not likely to increase patient participation in the care plan, but it should result in fewer medication errors for a number of reasons. It should eliminate handwritten orders, which are often illegible, and should trigger alerts to physicians if drug-drug interactions could occur or if there are medication overlaps or a need for corollary orders. The system should be able to automatically calculate doses according to the patient's criteria. Pharmacy response time should be faster.

**72. B:** If review of patients' EHRs shows that free text documentation by physicians describing patient conditions appears to be identical on consecutive days and on multiple patients' records, the most likely reason for this finding is that physicians are copying and pasting text. This is a common practice but can have serious repercussions because copied material may be inaccurate for the patient, and information in a patient's chart must be verified individually to ensure accurate reporting and billing.

**73. A:**

| Emp_ID | Last_Name | First_Name | Cred | Committee |
|--------|-----------|------------|------|-----------|
| 001 | James | Al | RPT | Health |
| 002 | Logan | Seth | RN | Telecom. |
| 003 | Roos | Linda | RN | Leisure |
| 004 | Davidson | Estella | LVN | Telecom. |

In the table above in a relational database, if the "Leisure" committee is discontinued and deleted from the database, Linda Roos (and any other members of the leisure committee as well) will be deleted from the database because of a deletion anomaly. A deletion anomaly occurs when deleting one type of data results in the unintended deletion of other data.

**74. C:** If a newer version of the software currently running the EHR has been issued, the type of testing that is usually indicated when a new version of software is issued and will be uploaded into the system is non-regression testing to determine if the software does what it is intended to do. Regression testing is often done with brand new software to determine if it causes errors or regressions as new software may adversely affect other parts of the system.

**75. B:** In order to submit immunization data electronically to an immunization registry, the organization must first have CEHRT (Certified electronic health record technology). CEHRT ensures that data are stored in a structured format and are secure. If the EHR meets criteria and is on the Certified Health IT Product List (CHPL) for certification, the healthcare organization must obtain a CMS EHR Certification ID from the Office of the National Coordinator of Health Information Technology (ONC).

**76. D:** During registration, a patient must sign an *assignment of benefits* form so that the provider can bill the insurance companies and receive reimbursement for claims directly. If there is no assignment of benefits, then the patient files the claim with the insurance company rather than the provider. This is sometimes the case if a patient is seeing a physician that is not in his/her network and doesn't, therefore, bill the insurance for care provided.

**77. A:** Under ICD-10-CM, external cause code reporting may be required by some states or payers but is otherwise voluntary and not mandatory. External cause codes are external or environmental causes of injury, such as "V90, Drowning and submersion due to accident to watercraft." Organizations are encouraged to voluntarily provide the information because these data provide valuable insight into the causes of injuries. These data are used to determine injury risk and to carry out research about preventive measures.

**78. C:** The Joint Commission (TJC) introduced the ORYX initiative in 1997 for the accreditation process in order to integrate outcomes data and performance measures. Requirements may vary somewhat from year to year. As of 2016, acute care hospitals are required to report on six sets of measures and critical access hospitals on four sets of measures. TJC provides chart-abstracted measure data and hospital performance data to hospitals based on reported information. The data are used to support benchmarking, standardization, and use of evidence-based care.

**79. A:** If during a recent outbreak of SARS, 86 patients were hospitalized with severe complications and 18 patient died in a 30-day period in which 26 patients died of other causes as well, the case fatality rate, rounded to the nearest whole number is 21%. When calculating the case fatality rate, the numerator is the number of cause-specific deaths (so other deaths are discounted), and the denominator is the number of patients diagnosed with the disease:

$$\frac{18}{86} \times 100\% = 0.2093 \times 100\% = 20.93\% \rightarrow 21\%$$

**80. B:** Hospitals may receive Medicare outlier payments for patient care cases with exceptionally high cost as a means to prevent hospitals from experiencing excessive financial losses for complex cases. In most cases, outlier payments account for 2 to 3% of IPPS payments although some hospitals may have higher rates. Certain high-risk procedures, such as solid organ transplants and tracheostomy with mechanical ventilation, are more likely to trigger outlier payments. CMS applies a formula with hospital-specific criteria to determine the amount of payment.

**81. D:** If a hospital has received a court order requesting documents from a patients' EHR for an attorney representing a patient in a negligence claim and the hospital attorney has also requested a copy of the records, only records specifically requested should be provided. Other records should not be provided unless they are covered in the court order. Records must be presented in exactly the same format to both attorneys. While it is not required to provide records in the PDF format, many facilities choose to provide documents in this form because the file can be easily duplicated to ensure all parties have the same exact copy.

**82. A:** Targeted efforts should be made to decrease actual ALOS for MS-DRG 61. While the weighting is highest (2.6877), patients with MCC are more costly to care for, and the patients average 8.67 days $(9 + 7 + 10 = 26/3)$. Since the GLOS (which eliminates outliers) is 5.4 and ALOS is 7.1, the actual average ALOS exceeds both. The actual average ALOS for MS-DRG 62 is 4 $(4 + 3 + 5 = 12/3)$ and for 63 is 3 $(4 + 2 + 4 + 2)$. Both of these averages are within the range of the MS-DRGs GLOS and ALOS.

**83. C:** When beginning the design of workload distribution for a distributed database, the initial step should be to analyze system and data storage requirements. Then, the global scheme is outlined followed by the designs for data distribution. In a distributed database, decisions must be made about how data are distributed across various sites in a network. Data are fragmented, partitioned into fragments that are allocated to different sites for storage. Fragmentation may be horizontal or vertical.

**84. D:** If a patient is admitted to an acute care hospital on September 6 and discharged on September 18, the Medicare benefit period ends 60 days in a row after discharge (counting the day of discharge) on November 16. Patients may have multiple stays in a hospital during one benefit period but may have only 90 days of hospitalization during one benefit period although each person has a once-in-a-lifetime 60-day extension that can be used for extended hospitalization.

**85. C:** Following a Medicare qualifying stay in an acute care hospital, a patient may be qualified for additional care in a skilled nursing facility (SNF) after discharge from the acute care hospital if admission to the SNF occurs within 30 days. The patient is covered for a stay not to exceed 100 days per benefit period. Payment is in full for the first 20 days only. After that, the patient has a daily co-payment.

**86. B:** If a healthcare provider has accepted assignment for services covered under Medicare, the healthcare provider agrees to accept the allowed charge as payment in full. Medicare, which is an 80-20 plan, pays 80% of usual, customary, and reasonable (UCR) charges, but payment varies from one area to another depending on a number of different factors. Many patients have supplemental insurance plans to cover the charges in excess of those allowed by Medicare.

**87. A:** Hardcoding of the chargemaster, linking services in the chargemaster to the correct CPS/HCPCS codes ensures that the services are charged for consistently. Hardcoding is typically used for professional services, such as laboratory services, respiratory therapy, and ECGs but not for room charges. With hardcoding, the code is generated when the charge is made rather than assigned at a later time by a coder. This practice can improve the revenue cycle because there is no delay in charging for services. Hardcoded services are those that generally do not change.

**88. A:** If the volume of patients in outpatient services has increased by 20% over the previous year, but a review of the revenue shows that medications and services typically provided to outpatients had decreased by 12%, resulting in a loss of revenue, the probable reason for this discrepancy is failure to code for services. The charges should be carefully audited to determine if a pattern emerges. For example, Medicare pays separately for injectable medications and administration, and the administration charge may be overlooked.

**89. B:** Prior to a facility carrying out diagnostic studies to be billed to Medicare, the healthcare provider must document medical necessity. This is done by applying the appropriate diagnostic coding to the order. If multiple tests are ordered, in some cases the order must contain multiple diagnostic codes. Some types of tests, such as those for research only or tests that are not FDA approved are not covered by Medicare, and the patient must, therefore, sign an Advance Beneficiary Notice.

**90. D:** If a healthcare provider has submitted a claim to Medicare under the Outpatient Prospective Payment System (OPPS), and outpatient code edits (OCE) indicate that there is a diagnosis code for vaginal bleeding during the first trimester of pregnancy but the gender selected is male (edit #3, diagnosis and sex conflict), the claim-level disposition that the healthcare provider should expect is the claim returned to the provider so that the problems can be corrected prior to resubmitting the claim.

**91. B:** If the HIM director has been assigned the position of chief compliance officer after a number of fraudulent practices in claims was identified, the first action of the compliance officer should be to review and reissue written standards of conduct, policies, and procedures. Fraudulent practices are not always intentional, and staff may need further ongoing education and training. A hotline can allow for anonymous complaints, and a system should be in place to respond to improper activity. Audits should be conducted routinely.

**92. A:** *Upcoding* occurs when a healthcare provider assigns a diagnosis or procedure code that will provide a higher return that the appropriate code. This may occur, for example, if a healthcare provider billed for a complete physical examination for a diagnosis of pneumonia but, in fact, only spent a few minutes with the patient who had a mild upper respiratory infection. Other fraudulent practices include unbundling (applying multiple codes in order to make several claims for what should be one inclusive code and service) and double billing, billing twice for the same service.

**93. C:** The tool by which the National Committee for Quality Assurance (NCQA) compares the quality of patient care provided by different health plans is HEDIS. HEDIS comprises 81 measures and 5 domains of care and is used by 9 out of 10 insurance companies to measure performance. HEDIS collects de-identified data directly from HMO and PPOs as well as Medicare and Medicaid. NCQA allows researchers access to the data so they can study trends in healthcare.

**94. A:** This information would be found in the physician's orders. While patient records may vary somewhat from one institution to another, the health record typically includes an admission form with demographic information, history and physical exam report, physician's orders, progress notes (physician, nurse, and other healthcare practitioners as indicated), laboratory reports, pathology reports (if appropriate), medication and treatment records, operative report (if indicated), consultant reports, and discharge summary.

**95. B:** The term used to describe a patient's age, weight, gender, pulse, and blood pressure is data elements as these are a series of single facts about the patient. Data (facts) that have been combined and analyzed or interpreted in some manner are classified as information. Data that are combined from various sources, such as from multiple patient's health records, is classified as aggregate data. Aggregate data are more easily obtained from EHRs than from paper records.

**96. D:** Information in the disease index is considered patient-identifiable data because the disease index links to the EHR by the patient's ID number, which is always included in the disease index. The disease index lists the disease codes (ICD-10-CM) for patients who are discharged. The disease index may contain various other information, such as the name of the patient's physician and the date of discharge.

**97. C:** When setting up a disease registry from existing data, the first step is to develop a case definition. The case definition establishes the guidelines for the information that will be included in the registry. For example, the case definition may be all patients with a specific diagnostic code, or it may be even more limited according to age, gender, or co-morbidities. It's important that the case definition remain consistent over the course of the registry or comparing data may be meaningless.

**98. A:** Metformin is a medication frequently used to treat diabetes mellitus, type 2 (E11) and this diagnostic information is missing. Medications and treatments indicated on the discharge summary should be linked to a diagnosis. Chronic conditions may be overlooked because if they are not the focus of care. In this case, the metoprolol is used to treat both primary hypertension and tachycardia. The hydrochlorothiazide is a diuretic used to control hypertension, and acetaminophen to control the pain of osteoarthritis.

**99. A:** If the hospital administration wants to develop a facility-specific cancer registry, the HIM director should recommend the discharge summary and disease index as the best sources for case finding. Once a case definition is established, coders can identify cases when reviewing the discharge data, and cases can be pulled from the disease index. The cancer registry may be used to assess mortality rates and treatment effectiveness and to facilitate patient follow-up after discharge.

**100. C:** If a patient suffered a severe reaction when administered the wrong drug and the director of risk management needs a complete description of the incident, the best source of information is the incident report. Incident reports are usually maintained separately from other records, and descriptions of errors in the EHR may be quite limited. That is, the medication and dosage may be recorded as well as the adverse effects, but not the fact that the medication was given in error.

**101. A:** If a medical scribe is used to enter documentation into the EHR for a physician, the individual who has the most responsibility to ensure that the EHR is complete and accurate is the attending physician. The physician should review the scribe-entered information and verify that it is correct. The physician is always most responsible for the health record. The HIM department reviews the record to assist the physician by pointing out deficiencies or errors.

**102. B:** When reviewing orders for medications, the RHIT, should be concerned if a physician has written the following order: Amlodipine 10.0 mg PO. The trailing zero (.0) should not be utilized as the period (.) could be overlooked and the dosage read as 100 mg. The Joint Commission has developed a "Do Not Use" list that applies to all hand-written/free text orders for medications and documentation of medication-related information. Other restrictions include the use of "MS" instead of morphine sulfate, the abbreviation "u" for unit, "IU" for international unit, QD, and QOD (or variations).

**103. D:** Assuming that all four elements in a row must be met to meet the criteria for the type of history, a visit with a patient for which the physician documented the chief complaint, an extended review of systems, and a pertinent past, family, and/or social history would not qualify as an E/M service because only 3 of 4 elements were met. The physician should be contacted to determine if the physician actually completed a history of present illness and simply failed to document it and, if so, whether it was brief or extended. If the physician failed to complete the history of the present illness, then the visit cannot be coded as an E/M service.

**104. C:** If the HIM contracts with a private agency to destroy paper health records that have been stored for over 10 years, assuming there are no specific state laws to the contrary, the contract should contain the destruction method, the duration of time between acquisition of the records and actual destruction, security measures to prevent breach, provisions for loss if unauthorized disclosure occurs, and details of liability insurance, including specified amounts. It is not necessary to include the inclusive dates of records although the hospital should include that information in its documentation.

**105. C:** SNOMED CT (Systemized Nomenclature of Medicine Clinical Terminology) is a reference terminology that provides a standardized vocabulary for medical conditions. SNOMED was developed by the College of American Pathologists. SNOMED CT is a designated standard for the exchange of electronic health information. A standardized vocabulary is critical for exchange of information and research. SNOMED CT references other terminologies and classification systems (such as ICD-10-CM) through cross mapping, which helps to reduce costs and minimize errors.

**106. D:** Three injury extensions are used with ICD-10-CM coding:

A: Initial encounter, such as the first visit to the emergency room for a fractured wrist when the patient is receiving active care for an injury.

D: Subsequent encounter, such as when the patient returns to the emergency room to have the cast removed or for other routine care

S: Sequela: Replaces "late effects" in ICD-9-CM and is used with complications that arise because of the initial injury, such as chronic nerve pain.

**107. A:** With ICD-10-PCS, the term *anastomosis* is not a root operation because it is integral to another procedure, such as a bypass operation. The root operation is the objective of the medical or surgical procedure. There are 31 root operations that are separated into 9 different groups depending on the function, including removal of a body part; removing solids/fluids/gasses from a body part; cutting or separating, moving or replacing some/part of a body part, altering the diameter/route of a tubular body part, using a device, examination only, other repairs, and other objectives. Multiple codes may be assigned.

**108. B:** As part of denials management, back-end editing is utilized to identify patient accounts that may not demonstrate medical necessity. A software application is used to scan the codes and look for discrepancies or problems indicating that the claim does not meet the criteria for medical necessity before the file is sent for billing so that the file can be reviewed again and corrections or additions requested. This approach can be used to reduce denials and improve cash flow.

**109. D:** If the registration clerk at one facility in a health information organization mistakenly pulls up a record from the master patient index (MPI) for a person with a similar name and demographic information when registering a patient for a procedure, this type of error is referred to as an overlap because one MPI entry (identifier) contains the records of two different people. Overlays may also occur if two records are accidentally merged.

**110. B:** When an unlisted procedure code is utilized under CPT coding, further documentation is required to support the claim. For laboratory tests, submissions include clinical notes that contain the patient's diagnosis as well as the name of the test and the test results. Unlisted procedure codes often end with "99." If an unlisted procedure code is utilized for a surgical procedure, then a copy of the operative report is required as an additional submission.

**111. A:** With CPT coding, if both a CPT modifier code and an HCPSC level II modifier code are utilized with a surgical procedure, the CPT modifier code is always placed in the first position and the HCPSC level II code in the second. Modifiers are always two-character codes and are utilized to add information to the original procedure code. The first modifier is most important because it may affect pricing. Modifiers may increase or reduce reimbursement.

**112. C:** If a patient underwent a major surgical procedure, such as an aortic aneurysm repair, the total number of days included in the global surgical package under Medicare guidelines is 92 days. One day preoperative is included as well as the day of surgery and the 90 days immediately following the procedure. These guidelines apply in any setting, so all routine care and necessary services provided during this time period are included as part of the package.

**113. A:** If a patient was scheduled for a bilateral simple complete mastectomy, but part way through the surgery, the patient developed severe cardiac dysrhythmias that could not be stabilized, so the surgery was discontinued, the incision closed, and the patient sent to the cardiac care unit, the correct CPT code is 19303-50-53. The first part (19303) is the planned procedure. This is followed by 50 to show that the procedure was bilateral. The code 53 indicates that the surgery was discontinued.

**114. C:** The purpose of the recovery audit contractor (RAC) program is to identify improper Medicare payments. Under the Tax Relief and Health Care Act (2006), the RAC program was made permanent after trial periods showed that it saved millions of dollars. The two types of audits conducted by RACs are automated reviews and complex reviews. Complex reviews are conducted manually and are used to target claims with a high likelihood of claims for non-covered services.

**115. C:** Eighteen shelving units are needed. If the bookcase units are 48 inches wide with 6 shelves per unit, this equals 288 inches of space ($48 \times 6 = 288$). Since there are 10,080 records with an average width of one-half inch ($10,080 \times 0.5$), 5040 inches of bookshelf are needed. By dividing the needed space by the total space in each bookshelf, the number of shelving units can be determined ($5040/288 = 17.5 \rightarrow 18$ units).

**116. D:** If the HIM department has used document imaging to archive medical records, the imaged records will provide access to patient records, but they are much more limited in scope than an EHR because they cannot capture discrete data elements, which might be desired for research. The imaged records are generally not immediately accessible but may take from one to 24 hours to access. The imaged records cannot be utilized for decision support, and they don't support alerts.

**117. C:** *Data granularity* is the characteristic of data quality that refers to the use of the specific level of detail required for a data element, such as ensuring three decimal spaces for the laboratory test of specific gravity (1.021). *Data definition* refers to the exact meaning of a data element. *Data currency* is the extent to which data is up-to-date. *Data precision* is how clearly the data values support the purpose.

**118. B:** Under PQRS (Physician Quality Reporting System) Measure #46, Medication Reconciliation, this crosscutting measure must be completed and reported for outpatient visits occurring within 30 days of discharge from an inpatient facility. Outpatient visits are classified as face-to-face encounters, such as office visits and outpatient visits, but do not include telehealth visits. This measure must be reported for two groups, (1) 18 to 64 years and (2) 65 and older. At least one cross-cutting measure must be reported for eligible professionals with face-to-face encounters.

**119. C:** The Credentialing and Re-credentialing Committee in an organization is usually not responsible for verifying an individual's credit history. The committee should focus on professional standards, such as whether licensure/credentialing is current, proof of liability insurance (including any liability claims history over a specified period of time), and completion of appropriate education (school, internship, residency) with verifying transcripts. Applicants for a new position are usually required to complete a questionnaire for the committee, including questions about illegal drug use and loss of license or felony convictions.

**120. A:** If the HIM department has received a request from an insurance carrier for a large number of different patient records for claims that do not appear to be problematical, the HIM department should question the reason for the requests before sending any records. For each request, the insurance company should explain the reason for the request, how the information will be used, and if any further disclosures will be made.

**121. D:** The fifth character in the ICD-10-PCS codes represents the medical and surgical approach used for a procedure. In this case, 0FT40ZZ (open cholecystectomy) is the correct answer because the fifth character is 0. Other codes include 3 (percutaneous), 4 (percutaneous endoscopic), 7 (via natural or artificial opening), 8 (via natural or artificial opening endoscopic), F (via natural or artificial opening with percutaneous endoscopic assistance, and X (external).

**122. B:** If a patient is severely allergic to penicillin and a controlled terminology that lists ingredients is used for the CPOE, the code that is most likely to trigger an alarm any time a penicillin drug is ordered is:

If ORDER = {any ingredient of ordered drug} = {any ingredient of allergic drug} then print "Alert!"

This same code should trigger an alert if any other drug to which the patient is allergic is ordered.

**123. C:** If an adult hospital wants to meet Leapfrog Group's standards for CPOE, 75% of physician orders must be made with a CPOE system that contains error-prevention software. An additional requirement is that the hospital must conduct tests that show that physicians are alerted to common prescribing errors at least 50% of the time. Leapfrog Group is a voluntary program that promotes quality in healthcare, safety, and affordability and applies letter grades (A-F) to participating hospitals.

**124. A:** If County Hospital accepts credit card payments, it must comply with security controls set by PCI DSS (Payment Card Industry Data Security Standard). There are 5 audit requirements:

A process must be in place to link all access done through administrative privileges (root access) to individual users.

Automated audit trails should be implemented to track a number of different events, such as access to cardholder data.

Audit trails must record at least user identification, event type, date, time, success/failure of query, origination, and identify/name of data, component, or resource affected.

Audit trails must not be alterable.

Logs of system components must be reviewed daily.

**125. C:** For the HHS Office of Civil rights (OCR) HIPAA audits, scheduled to begin in 2016, the three compliance categories are:

Security: Organizations should complete a security risk assessment.

Privacy: HIPAA policy requirements for privacy should be reviewed as well as how PHI is used and disclosed. Policies regarding training, disciplinary actions as well as security management should be reviewed.

Breach notification: Policies regarding how the organization deals with breaches and who needs to be organized should be reviewed and updates.

**126. B:** Data mapping:

| ICD-9-CM | Description | ICD-10-CM | Description | Approx. | No map |
|---|---|---|---|---|---|
| E850.0 | Accidental poisoning by heroin | | | 0 | 1 |
| E851 | Accidental poisoning by barbiturates | | | 0 | 1 |

Based on the General Equivalence Mapping above, the ICD-9-CM codes E850.0 (accidental poisoning by heroin) and E851 (accidental poisoning by barbiturates) cannot be mapped to ICD-10-CM codes, as there is no direct or approximate equivalent.

**127. B:** With ICD-10-PCS, if a patient's gastrostomy tube develops a leak and is removed and a new gastrostomy tube placed into the same opening, the root operation utilized for this procedure is *change*. *Replacement* is used when a body part is removed and replaced with synthetic material, such as a hip replacement. *Insertion* is placing a non-biological device, such as a radioactive implant, into a body part to monitor, assist, or prevent a physiological function. *Revision* involves correcting a malfunctioning or displaced device, such as a pacemaker.

**128. B:** When preparing for an external coding audit, the HIM director should avoid advising coders that the outcomes will be used for disciplinary actions. Rather, the HIM director should stress the positive aspects of an audit and should communicate the goals of the process before the audit begins. The HIM director should stress the educational advantage to the external coding audit and work with individual coding professionals to establish performance goals.

**129. A:** A "never event" is one that should never occur in a healthcare setting, such as if a patient scheduled for a cholangiogram underwent a colonoscopy in error. The three primary types of never events include (1) carrying out the wrong operation or procedure on the correctly identified patient, (2) carrying out the wrong operation or procedure on an incorrectly identified (wrong) patient, and (3) carrying out the correct operation or procedure on the wrong body site/part on a correctly identified patient.

**130. B:** In terms of filing claims, "bundling" refers to including a number of different procedures under one code. This is commonly done, for example, when the same steps are taken time for a surgical procedure. Bundling saves time when it comes to coding. In some cases, such as when an unusual event occurs during a bundled procedure, unbundling may be done, but if unbundling is done just to increase payments, then it is a fraudulent practice.

**131. A:** Ambulance service requires a HCPCS level II code for a CMS claim. HCPCS level I comprises CPT codes while HCPCS level II comprises services that are not included in the CPT codes. Others examples of supplies, services or products covered by HCPCS level II codes include durable medical equipment, orthotics, and prostheses. There are four types of HCPCS level II codes: permanent national codes, dental codes, miscellaneous codes, and temporary national codes.

**132. C:** For claims for durable medical equipment, prosthetics, orthotics, and supplies (DMEPOS) for which no code currently exists, the organization filing the claim should first contact the DME MACs PDAC (pricing, data, and analysis contractor). The PDAC can help in determining which

HCPCS code is most appropriate and can provide guidance regarding appropriate supporting documentation. The PDAC may assign a miscellaneous code or a non-covered item/service code. The PDAC also has a product classification list available online.

**133. A:** If a patient had a kidney removed for "renal cell carcinoma," the RHIT would use the "Malignant primary" column on the ICD-10-CM Table of Neoplasms to identify the correct code as a renal cell carcinoma in the kidney would be a primary lesion. The terms "carcinoma" and "sarcoma" either by themselves, such as in "renal carcinoma," or combined, such as in "osteosarcoma" refer to malignant neoplasms.

**134. C:** A complete NDC consists of 3 different sub-codes:

Labeler code: The firm that manufactures, re-packages, or distributes, supplied to the firm by the FDA.

Product code: The code identifying the drug and dosage, supplied by the firm.

Package code. The code identifying the size and type of package, supplied by the firm.

Code configuration (in digits) may be 4-4-2, 5-3-2, 5-4-1, or 5-4-2, but CMA follows the HIPAA standard of 5-4-2 (11 digits) and uses leading zeroes for shorter codes.

**135. B:** The primary purpose of the RxNorm dose form is to describe the form in which a drug is presented. This does not necessarily reflect the way the drug is administered. Example:

| Form | Definition & Usage Notes |
|---|---|
| Foam | Bubble of gas that are introduced into a liquid |
| Injectable foam | A foam intended to be injected |
| Oral foam | A foam intended to be administered into the mouth |
| Rectal foam | A foam intended for use in the rectum |

Source: National Library of Medicine.

**136. D:** LOINC (Logical Observation Identifiers, Names, and Codes) provides a set of identifiers and names for observations, such as laboratory data and clinical data. LOINC is maintained by a non-profit organization, the Regenstrief Institute. LOINC is used with EHRs and is a US government standard for the exchange of electronic health information. LOINC is especially useful for the exchange of information from one system to another. Each test/observation is covered by six fields in the database: component, kind of property, aspect of time, system, scale type, and method type.

**137. A:** If a database provides an alert when a patient's birthdate entered into a field shows that a patient being admitted for delivery of an infant is four years old, this type of validation is a consistency check. A consistency check compares data in two different fields to determine if the values entered are reasonable. A consistency check cannot identify all errors and is limited by parameters that are set for the fields and for the validation.

**138. A:** Coordination of Benefits (COB) is the process that ensures when claims are filed with Medicare and secondary insurers that the primary insurer is identified as well as secondary insurers and the extent of their contributions. COB information can be obtained through IRS/SSA/CMS Claims Data Match, Voluntary Data Sharing Agreements (VDSAs), COBA program, Initial Enrollment Questionnaire (IEQ), Section 111 of the MMSEA, and other data exchanges.

**139. D:** In order to receive Meaningful Use payments, an organization must carry out a risk analysis to determine if there are security risks that may result in a security breach of PHI. Once a risk analysis has identified areas of potential security breaches, then the organization must take the steps necessary to secure PHI and must document and provide evidence of compliance to CMS. While 100% security is the aim, it is not always possible to absolutely ensure 100% security.

**140. C:** According to HIPAA's Privacy Rule, diagnoses do not have to be removed when de-identifying data as diagnoses are essential for research purposes. Elements that must be removed include names, dates (except year) directly related to the individual (such as birthdate, date of death), identifying numbers (medical record, FAZ, email addresses, health plan, account, certificate/license, vehicle identifier, device identifier, and IP address), identifying geographic information, biometric information, full face photographic images, and comparable images.

**141. D:** In the revenue cycle, "charge capture" refer to charges converted to billable fees. This conversion takes place either manually, electronically, or some combination and is dependent of appropriate and accurate coding. Healthcare organizations are under increasing pressure to capture all charges because significant loss occurs when charges are not billed, a problem that is especially common with outpatient services. Formal accountability measures that include ongoing evaluation is critical to adequate charge capture.

**142. B:** TRICARE Extra is the least expensive TRICARE option and is a paid provider organization. TRICARE Extra requires that enrollees choose a physician from among those on a provider list. TRICARE Extra is available to retired service members and their families and the families of active duty service members but is not an option for those in active duty. Enrollees must pay an annual deductible (sponsor rank E4 and below $50 per person, $100 per family; sponsor rank E5 and above, $150 per person and $300 per family) and make copayments, but there is no enrollment fee or annual fee.

**143. B:** The three levels of severity in the MS-DRG system are MCC (major complications/co-morbidities), CC (complications/co-morbidities), and Non-CC (no complications/comorbidities). These levels are based on secondary diagnoses. For example, if a patient has open heart surgery, the MS-DRG would be assigned for that primary diagnosis; however, if the patient developed sepsis, the level of severity would be assigned based on the secondary diagnosis of sepsis.

**144. C:** MS-DRG adjustments to base rate are not made based on transfer policy although the transfer policy affects the amount of payment each facility receives. MS-DRG adjustments are made based on 4 criteria:

Value based purchasing: increase or decrease depending on positive or negative VBP.

Hospital readmission reduction program: Increase or decrease depending on whether hospital readmissions are decreased or not.

Disproportionate share hospitals: Increased payments for hospitals with disproportionate share of low-income patients.

Indirect medical education: Increased payment for teaching hospitals.

**145. D:** If a physician on staff at County Hospital requests copies of his sister's health records following her hospitalization for an MI, the appropriate response is to refuse the request because allowing him unauthorized access to PHI is a HIPAA violation. The sister can request copies of the health record and allow the physician to look at the records, or the sister can grant the physician power of attorney so that he can legally request the records.

**146. C:** If a patient is being treated for recent onset of depression (F06.31) associated with uncontrolled hypothyroidism due to atrophy of the thyroid gland (E03.4), the primary diagnosis is hypothyroidism because it is the underlying cause of the depression. Since the patient is currently still receiving treatment for hypertension (I10), that code would come next. The last code is the history of malignancy (Z85). The code sequence is: E03.4, F06.31, I10, and Z85.

**147. D:** If County Hospital has an average cost per patient day of $2000 and a CMI of 1.10, its adjusted cost per patient day is $1818.18 (2000/1.10). A CMI higher than 1.0 results in decreased cost per patient and a CMI lower than 1.0 results in increased cost per patient. Generally the higher the CMI, but better off the hospital is financially, so any drop in CMI should be rigorously evaluated to determine what measure can be taken to increase the CMI.

**148. A:** If a patient has undergone ambulatory surgery and the physician has written "suspected cholelithiasis" as the first-listed diagnosis on the front sheet of the patient's record, in order to code the first-listed diagnosis correctly, the coding professional should review the operative report for the diagnosis. If a preoperative diagnosis and a postoperative diagnosis differ, then the post-operative diagnosis should be coded. Codes should never be assigned to diagnoses that are qualified ("suspected").

**149. D:** If an RHIT conducting a record analysis notes that a patient's health record is missing the *Consent for Operation and/or Procedures*, the RHIT should notify a supervisor who can address the issue. The physician who performed the operation/procedure without assuring a consent was formed should receive appropriate education. A consent form cannot be signed and added to a record after the fact, and if for some reason a procedure was performed without consent (such as in an emergent situation), then the reason should be fully documented.

**150. A:** Before assigning an APC (Ambulatory Payment Classification) code to a claim for an outpatient procedure in an ambulatory surgery center, the coding professional must first assign as ICD-10-CM diagnostic code and a CPT/HCPCS procedure code. Software applications are usually used to indicate the correct APC for a CPT code. Outpatient PPS payment is based on the APC system, which includes procedural groups with procedures that are similar and require similar resources. The rates vary according to geographical area and are wage adjusted.

**151. A:** Accounts Receivable (A/R) management is the process by which outstanding accounts are monitored to facilitate timely reimbursement. Outstanding accounts are those charges for which a patient or payer have failed to reimburse the healthcare organization. The A/R ratio shows the percentage of outstanding charges compared to total charges:

$$A/R = \text{Total charges} - \text{net collections}$$
$$= 132{,}000 - 92{,}000$$
$$= 40{,}000$$

$$A/R \text{ ratio} = \frac{A/R}{\text{average monthly charges}}$$
$$= \frac{40{,}000}{128{,}000}$$
$$= 0.3125 \rightarrow 31.25\%$$

**152. C:** If the HIM director is managing a project to upgrade the HIM system, the three project cost management processes the director must carry out are:

Estimating costs: Includes development of activity cost estimates, basis of estimates, and project document updates as well as development of a cost management plan.

Establishing the budget: Includes allocation of funds and development of a cost performance baseline, funding requirements, and project document updates.

Controlling costs: Includes constant monitoring of work performance, measures, and budget forecasts.

**153. B:** If a large hospital has the same coders coding both inpatient and outpatient records and a coding audit shows increasing numbers of errors in coding over the previous 6 months, the best solution may be to change to coding specialization, with some coders working only on inpatient records and some only on outpatient records. Because there are significant differences between the two types of records and the coding requirements, specialization may improve performance.

**154. B:** If a physician at an ambulatory surgery center carries out a procedure normally done only as an inpatient and the OPPS status indicator for the HCPCS/CPT code is "C," no reimbursement should be expected. A "C" status indicator means that the procedure must be done as an inpatient and should not have been done as an outpatient because of risks to the patient. This type of error should not occur because it indicates a failure to follow procedure in verifying codes.

**155. C:** According to the DRG data from the cardiac care unit, the code that has resulted in the highest reimbursement is 280, acute myocardial infarction discharged alive w MCC. Although this code has only the third highest number of discharges, because the relative weight is so high, the total weight is highest:

$$291: 1.4822 \times 1208 = 1790.4976$$
$$292: 0.9703 \times 2506 = 2431.5718$$
$$280: 1.6969 \times 1856 = 3132.4774$$
$$282: 0.7823 \times 2078 = 1625.6194$$

**156. A:** If a hospital had 826 discharges over a 30-day period and experienced 32 deaths, including 2 newborns, 4 children, and 3 adults who died within 48 hours of admission, the gross death rate (rounded to one decimal point for this period is 3.8%:

$$32/826 = 0.03847 = 0.038 \times 100 = 3.8\%$$

The *gross* death rate is the basic indicator of mortality used by healthcare facilities and includes all deaths (newborns, children, and adults) regardless of the amount of time that has passed since admission. The *net* death rate omits those who died within 48 hours of admission.

**157. D:** From an ethical perspective, the principle of *beneficence* is operational if the HIM professional releases information about a patient only with proper authorization and for the good of the patient. This may include releasing records to the patient so that the patient can monitor healthcare or to insurance companies so that claims can be reimbursed. Nonmaleficence is operational when the HIM professional checks authorization to make sure there is no unauthorized access. Justice is allowing all patients equal access, and autonomy is allowing the patient to make decisions about access to information.

**158. D:** A *potentially compensable event* is an incident that can lead to financial loss or legal action, such as a medicine or surgical error. When a potentially compensable event occurs, an incident report must be filed immediately by those involved in or witnessing the event. This incident report is filed separately from the health record. Risk management reviews potentially compensable events to determine liability issues and necessary actions to reduce risk.

**159. B:** If, a patient complained of pain in the right knee and a physician ordered an x-ray of the right knee, CBC, metabolic panel, and chest x-ray and the results showed an elevated white count of 10,000 and slightly elevated glucose (106), the coding professional should code M25.561, Pain in right knee, and query the physician regarding further diagnoses to explain the additional lab work and chest x-ray. The coder should never guess at a diagnosis or chose a diagnosis that supports medical necessity if the documentation in the patient's health record provides no supporting evidence.

**160. C:** If County hospital has experienced a recent increase in medical-necessity denials from Medicare, and the different levels of appeals and costs have negatively impacted the return on investment, the best place to begin to determine the cause of the denials and to take steps to remedy the situation is assessing denials data. Aggregate data can be pulled from EHRs and evaluated to determine if there are patterns that emerge to explain the increased rate of denials.

**161. B:** In a 30-day period, if 46 infants were discharged for NICU and 8 infants became infected as the result of an outbreak of Enterobacteriaceae in a 30-day period, the infection rate for that time period is 17.4%:

$$8/46 = 0.17391 = 1.74 \times 100 = 17.4\%$$

Hospitals routinely monitor hospital-acquired infection and postoperative infections rates as these must be reported. Infection rates in general should be monitored on at least a monthly basis, especially in high-risk areas, such as NICU and ICU.

**162. D:** If an outpatient radiological procedure with contrast resulted in a lump-sum payment for both the technical component of the procedure and the professional component, this type of payment is referred to as global payment. Global payments are commonly used for radiological and other similar outpatient services. The professional component involves injection of the contrast material and the technical component is the X-ray or CT. Global surgery payments may be paid in some instances as well.

**163. C:** According to NHIN, the three dimensions of infrastructure needed for HIM systems are:

Personal health dimension: Core content includes information from the personal health record, other elements (audit logs, advance directives), and elements from community health (living environment).

Healthcare provider dimension: Core content includes patient health record and supporting notes and laboratory findings, other elements (protocols, CDS programs), and elements from community health dimension (community health resources, environmental hazards).

Population health dimension: Core content includes public health data and other elements (de-identified health status/outcomes, community directories).

**164. B:** If a patient of a home health agency required only 4 visits in a 60-day period, this will trigger a low-utilization payment adjustment (LUPA), with payments made according to the number of visits. The reimbursement rate is higher rate than standard payment for initial LUPA visits that are limited to only the initial visit or to the initial visit of a sequence of adjacent visits. Partial-episode payment (PEP) is made if a patient transfers from one HHA to another in the midst of care or if the patient is discharged from care and then readmitted within a 60-day period.

**165. A:** If a patient was admitted to the hospital with a severe headache but the physician failed to order a head CT and discharged the patient who subsequently died with a subdural hemorrhage, the type of negligence that could be charged is nonfeasance, a failure to act in accordance to standard medical practice. In this case, the harm would be unintentional. This differs slightly from malfeasance, which is causing intentional injury, such as with the removal of the wrong body part. Misfeasance is unintentional injury that occurs as the result of a correct act, such as perforating the intestines during a colonoscopy.

# Thank You

We at Mometrix would like to extend our heartfelt thanks to you, our friend and patron, for allowing us to play a part in your journey. It is a privilege to serve people from all walks of life who are unified in their commitment to building the best future they can for themselves.

The preparation you devote to these important testing milestones may be the most valuable educational opportunity you have for making a real difference in your life. We encourage you to put your heart into it—that feeling of succeeding, overcoming, and yes, conquering will be well worth the hours you've invested.

We want to hear your story, your struggles and your successes, and if you see any opportunities for us to improve our materials so we can help others even more effectively in the future, please share that with us as well. **The team at Mometrix would be absolutely thrilled to hear from you!** So please, send us an email (support@mometrix.com) and let's stay in touch.

If you feel as though you need additional help, please check out the other resources we offer:

**Study Guide: http://MometrixStudyGuides.com/RHIT**

**Flashcards: http://MometrixFlashcards.com/RHIT**